The Anatomy of
Exercise & Movement

for the study of dance, pilates, sport and yoga

Jo Ann Staugaard-Jones

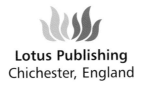

Lotus Publishing
Chichester, England

First published in 2010 by
Lotus Publishing
Apple Tree Cottage, Inlands Road, Nutbourne, Chichester, PO18 8RJ, UK

Disclaimer

This book is not meant as a substitute for medical advice. If you have any medical condition or if you experience pain or discomfort with the exercises contained within this book, then you must stop immediately and consult a qualified medical practitioner. Both the Publisher and the Author accept no responsibility for any consequences of the advice given if medical advice is not sought and followed before beginning a new exercise programme.

All Drawings Amanda Williams and Pascale Pollier
Text Design Wendy Craig
Cover Design Jim Wilkie
Printed and Bound in the UK by Scotprint

British Library Cataloguing in Publication Data
A CIP record for this book is available from the British Library
ISBN 978 1 905367 17 7

Distribution in UK/Europe
Combined Book Services Limited
Unit Y, Paddock Wood Distribution Centre
Paddock Wood
Tonbridge, Kent, TN12 6UU
Phone 01892 837171
Fax 01892 837272
orders@combook.co.uk

Distribution in North America
Cardinal Publishers Group
2402 Shadeland Avenue, Suite A
Indianapolis, IN 46219
Phone 317-352-8200
Fax 317-352-8202
customerservice@cardinalpub.com

Discount available for bulk orders.

Contents

Introduction 5

Chapter 1: Anatomical Direction, Planes and Movement 7
Terms to Describe Direction 8
Planes of the Body 9
Terms to Describe Movement 10

Chapter 2: Skeletal Muscle and Muscle Mechanics 13
The Physiology of Muscle Contraction .18
Muscle Reflexes 19
Musculo-skeletal Mechanics 20
Levers 22
Generation of Force 23
Muscles Involved in Breathing 24
Synovial Joints 25

Chapter 3: The Spine 27
The Vertebral Spine 29
Cervical Region 30
Cervical Muscles 31
Thoracic Region 35
Thoracic Muscles 36
Myths of the Upper Spine Dispelled 45
Main Muscles Involved in Movements of the Spine 46

Chapter 4: The Core 47
Lumbar Region 48
Lumbar Muscles 48
Abdominal Muscle #1: Rectus Abdominis 49
Abdominal Muscle #2: External Obliques 54
Abdominal Muscle #3: Internal Obliques 56
Abdominal Muscle #4: Transversus Abdominis 57
Psoas Major 63
Quadratus Lumborum 68
The Pelvis 69
Myths of the Core Dispelled 75
Main Muscles Involved in Movements of the Thoracic/Lumbar Spine 75

Chapter 5: The Shoulder Region 77
Glenohumeral Joint 78
Movements of the Shoulder Joint 79
Shoulder Joint Muscles 80
Deltoids 82
Pectoralis Major 84
Latissimus Dorsi 86
The Rotator Cuff 87
Shoulder Girdle Joint 91
Movements of the Shoulder Girdle 91
Shoulder Girdle Muscles 92
Trapezius 93
Summary: The Shoulder Joint and Girdle Combined 95
Myths of the Shoulder Dispelled 99
Main Muscles Involved in Movements of the Shoulder Region 100

Chapter 6: The Elbow and Radio-ulnar Joints 101
The Elbow Joint 102
Biceps Brachii 104
Triceps Brachii 105
Elbow Injuries 107
The Radio-ulnar Joint 108
Muscles of the Radio-ulnar Joint 109
Myths of the Elbow and Radio-ulnar Joints Dispelled 112
Main Muscles Involved in Movements of the Elbow and Radio-ulnar Joints 112

Chapter 7: The Wrist and Hand **113**
Muscles of the Wrist 117
Injuries/Conditions of the Wrist and Hand 117
Myths of the Wrist and Hand Dispelled 121
Main Muscles Involved in Movements of the Wrist, Hand, Fingers and Thumb 121

Chapter 8: The Iliofemoral (Hip) Joint **123**
Anterior Hip (Flexor) Muscles 124
Lateral Hip (Abductor) Muscles 131
Posterior Hip (Extensor) Muscles 139
The Iliofemoral ("Y") Ligament 142
Medial Hip (Adductor) Muscles 147
Six Deep Rotators 152
Inward Rotators of the Hip 155
Myths of the Iliofemoral (Hip) Joint Dispelled 157
Main Muscles Involved in Movements of the Iliofemoral (Hip) Joint 157

Chapter 9: The Knee Joint 159
Knee Extensors: Quadriceps Femoris 162
Knee Flexors: The Hamstrings 165
Knee Injuries 167
Myths of the Knee Dispelled 172
Main Muscles Involved in Movements of the Knee Joint 172

Chapter 10: The Ankle Joint and Foot **173**
Joints and Actions of the Ankle Joint and Foot 174
Muscles of the Ankle Joint and Foot 176
The Foot 181
Ligaments of the Ankle Joint and Foot 182
Ankle Joint and Foot Conditions 183
Myths of the Foot Dispelled 185
Main Muscles Involved in Movements of the Ankle Joint and Foot 186

Appendix: Jaw and Thoat 187
References 188
Index 189

Introduction

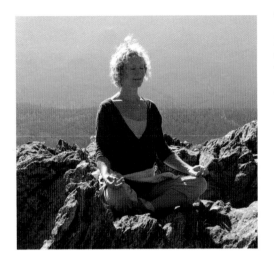

This is a book about muscles and movement. Chapters center on specific joint areas, relating them to current concepts and myths in an informative and useful way. Content includes detailed material on location and actions of different muscles, with descriptions and illustrations of strength and stretch exercises for each joint area. Exercises cover a wide scope of fitness areas: weight-training, yoga, pilates, dance, and sports.

The author at Shoshoni Yoga Retreat Center, Colorado.

The book's approach is unique because it can be used as a handbook, a resource for those who would like to know more about the human body without having to read a cumbersome textbook. The book is readable and interesting, for anyone from beginners, to teachers of movement, to a resource for exercise science and fitness enthusiasts and professionals.

There is a hunger for written material about movement that can be understood by a majority of the population. There are an increasing number of people who are interested in learning about their body, how it moves, and what can be done to improve it, without the fitness 'hype'. This book is a "kinesiology made easier" approach that is valid and needed. Many students and teachers desire a book that is precise yet understandable, and relates directly to their own lifestyle. This text does just that.

My motivation for composing such a book comes from my movement teaching experiences, listening to students and what they desire. My graduate education in Exercise Science and Dance has led to over 30 years of college teaching. My background in sports and dance along with certifications in Pilates and Yoga has resulted in a broad range of teaching material, and a love for working with those people who are serious about being naturally healthy.

I feel this book can be read and enjoyed by anyone interested in the human body and its potential. **Natural prevention is the key to a healthy body.**

Jo Ann Staugaard-Jones, 2010

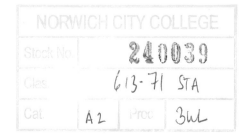

About the Author

Jo Ann Staugaard-Jones, professor and author, has taught movement workshops and master classes at universities such as Boston University, Colorado State University, Williams College, Cornell, Temple, University of Buffalo, Arizona State University, and Miami, as well as many Health Clubs, Yoga, and Pilates studios throughout the USA and abroad. She is a full professor of Dance and Kinesiology, a member of IADMS, the International Association of Dance Medicine & Science, a certified Shambhava Hatha Yoga Instructor, and a Power Pilates teacher. She received her undergraduate degree from Kansas University and her Master in Arts from New York University, and continues to reside in northwest New Jersey and Colorado. She is currently teaching interactive movement workshops across the US, and sponsors international holistic retreats through www.neatretreats.com.   She can be reached at jojones3@verizon.net.

Exercise Notes

The Anatomy of Exercise & Movement is designed to provide a balance of theoretical information about muscles and movement, and Chapters 3–10 focus on a specific joint(s). To complement the material written about each joint(s), there are a series of both strengthening and stretching exercises where appropriate, and technique instructions on how to perform each exercise. To visually help the reader fully understand the nuances and muscles involved, where possible, the exercise has been illustrated. The difficulty of each exercise is indicated by *I = beginning; II = intermediate; III = advanced*.

The muscle information given may be too much for some people or not enough for others, but hopefully will aid anyone who wants to tone or strengthen certain areas. If one knows where the muscle is located and what exercise works it, then a specific exercise program can be designed. Stretching is always a great way to begin a workout, with dynamic stretching being most effective. Static stretching is best at the end of a workout, to relax and lengthen muscles.

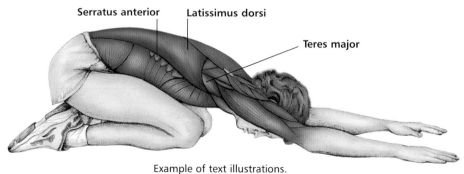

Example of text illustrations.

TECHNIQUE

Kneel on the ground and reach forward with hands. Let the head fall forward and push the buttocks toward feet.

Chapter 1

Anatomical Direction, Planes and Movement

The anatomical position provides a standard reference point for an individual, where the body is upright, head, eyes, and toes, all facing forward and with the arms and hands hanging by the sides, palms turned.

Terms to Describe Direction

Anterior. Situated or toward the front of the body. (Also called ventral.) So a term prefixed with antero- signifies before.
Posterior. Situated toward the back of the body (Also called dorsal.) Postero- is a combining form, denoting relationship to the posterior part, e.g. posterolateral.

Inferior. Situated below, or directed down, away from the head.
Superior. Situated above, toward the head.

Lateral. Toward the side of the body, or located away from the midline of the body or organ.
Medial. Toward the midline of the body or organ.
Peripheral. Toward the outer surface of the body or organ.

Distal. From the Latin, distans, meaning distant. Remote; away from any point of origin of a structure.
Proximal. From the Latin, proximus, meaning next. Nearest; closer to any point of origin of a structure.

Deep. Situated far from the body surface.
Superficial. Situated near or at the body surface.

Dorsum. The back, or posterior surface of something, e.g. back of the hand, or upper surface of the foot.
Palmar. The anterior surface of the hand.
Plantar. The sole of the foot.

Prone. Position of the body in which the ventral (anterior) surface faces down.
Supine. Position of the body in which the ventral (anterior) surface faces up.

Opposition. Movement of the thumb to approach or touch one or more of the fingertips.
Reposition. Returning the thumb to a parallel position with the fingers.

Ipsilateral. On the same side.
Contralateral. On the opposite side.

Planes of the Body

The mid-sagittal (sagitta is Latin for 'arrow') (or median) plane is a vertical plane extending in an anteroposterior direction dividing the body into right and left parts; effectively the forward and backward plane. (A sagittal plane is any plane parallel to the median plane.)

The coronal (or frontal) plane is a vertical plane at right angles to the sagittal plane that divides the body into anterior and posterior portions; effectively the side movement plane.

The transverse (or horizontal) plane is a horizontal cross-section, dividing the body into upper and lower sections, and lies at right angles to the other two planes; effectively the rotational movement plane.

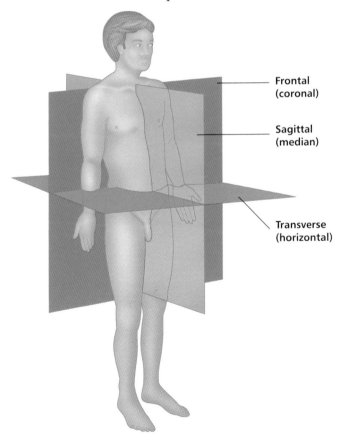

Frontal (coronal)

Sagittal (median)

Transverse (horizontal)

Planes of the body.

Each plane has specific joint actions. In the sagittal plane, the actions of flexion and extension happen. A good example of flexion is any movement that takes the body toward fetal position; extension is the return from flexion. In the frontal plane, generally abduction and adduction take place; 'jumping jacks' are an example of these two actions at the shoulder and hip joints. At the spine, the frontal actions are lateral flexion right and left (side bending). In the transverse plane, various forms of rotation happen, including internal and external rotation, pronation and supination, and upward and downward rotation, depending on the joint.

Terms to Describe Movement

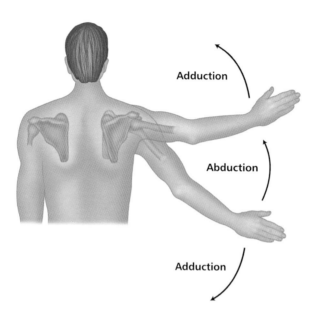

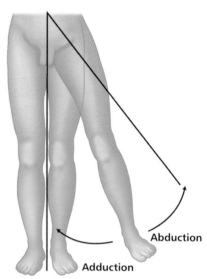

Abduction. Movement away from the midline of the body (or to return from adduction).

Adduction. Movement toward the midline of the body (or to return from abduction).

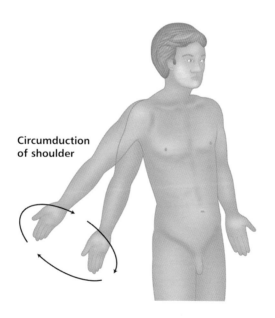

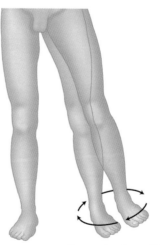

Circumduction of leg

Circumduction. Movement in which the distal end of a bone moves in a circle, whilst the proximal end remains relatively stable; combining flexion, extension, abduction and adduction.

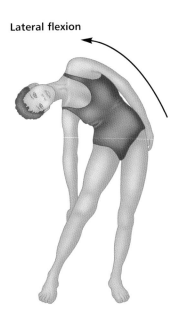

Lateral flexion

Lateral flexion. Bending the body or head sideways in the coronal plane.

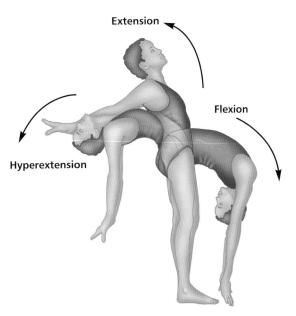

Extension

Hyperextension

Flexion

Extension. Movement that straightens or increases the angle between the bones or part of the body. (Hyperextension is extreme or excessive extension beyond the normal range.)

Flexion. Movement that involves bending, e.g. spine, bending forward.

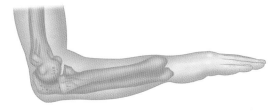

Pronation. Rotating the forearm to turn the palm of the hand down to face the floor, or to face posteriorly from the anatomical position.

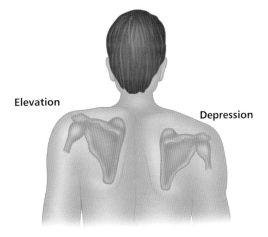

Elevation

Depression

Depression. Movement of an elevated part of the body downward to its original position.

Elevation. Movement of a part of the body upwards along the frontal plane.

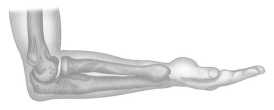

Supination. Rotating the forearm to turn the palm of the hand up to face the ceiling, or to face forward, as is the case in the anatomical position.

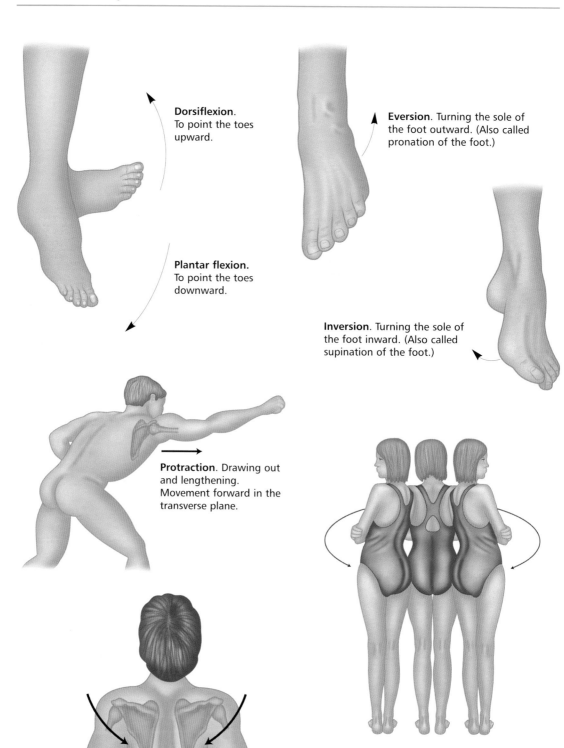

Dorsiflexion. To point the toes upward.

Plantar flexion. To point the toes downward.

Eversion. Turning the sole of the foot outward. (Also called pronation of the foot.)

Inversion. Turning the sole of the foot inward. (Also called supination of the foot.)

Protraction. Drawing out and lengthening. Movement forward in the transverse plane.

Rotation. Turning around a fixed axis. Medial rotation: Turning in toward the midline. Lateral rotation: Turning out away from the midline.

Retraction. Drawing back. Movement backward in the transverse plane.

Chapter

2

Skeletal Muscle and Muscle Mechanics

The human body contains over 215 pairs of skeletal muscles, which make up approximately 40% of its weight. Skeletal muscles are so named because most attach to and move the skeleton, and so are responsible for movement of the body.

Skeletal muscles have an abundant supply of blood vessels and nerves, which is directly related to contraction, the primary function of skeletal muscle. Each skeletal muscle generally has one main artery to bring nutrients via the blood supply, and several veins to take away metabolic waste.

The blood and nerve supply generally enters the muscle through the centre of the muscle, but occasionally toward one end, which eventually penetrates the endomysium around each muscle fiber.

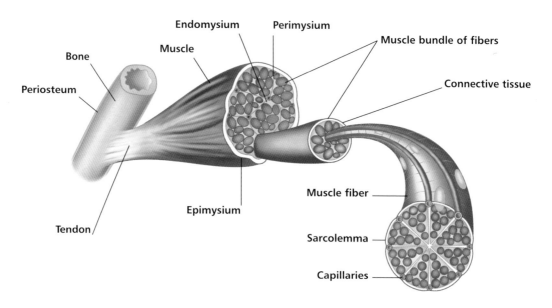

Figure 2.1: A cross-section of skeletal muscle tissue.

The three types of skeletal muscle fiber are: red slow-twitch, intermediate fast-twitch and white fast-twitch. The colour of each is reflected in the amount of myoglobin present, a store for oxygen. The myoglobin is able to increase the rate of oxygen diffusion, so red slow-twitch fibers are able to contract for longer periods, which is particularly useful for endurance events. The white fast-twitch fibers have a lower content of myoglobin. Because they rely on glycogen (energy) reserves, they can contract quickly, but they also fatigue quickly, so are more prevalent in sprinters, or sports where short, rapid movements are required, such as weightlifting. World-class marathon runners have been reported to possess 93-99% slow-twitch fibers in their gastrocnemius (calf) muscle, whilst world-class sprinters only possessed about 25% in the same muscle (Wilmore & Costill, 1994).

Each skeletal muscle fiber is a single cylindrical muscle cell, which is surrounded by a plasma membrane called the sarcolemma. The sarcolemma features specific openings, which lead to tubes known as transverse (or T) tubules. (The sarcolemma maintains a membrane potential, which allows impulses, specifically to the sarcoplasmic reticulum (SR), to either generate or inhibit contractions.)

An individual skeletal muscle may be made up of hundreds, or even thousands, of muscle fibers bundled together and wrapped in a connective tissue sheath called the epimysium, which gives the muscle its shape, as well as providing a surface against which the surrounding muscles can move. Fascia, connective tissue outside the epimysium, surrounds and separates the muscles.

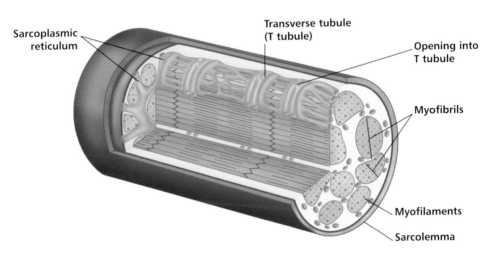

Figure 2.2: Each skeletal muscle fiber is a single cylindrical muscle cell.

Portions of the epimysium project inward to divide the muscle into compartments. Each compartment contains a bundle of muscle fibers; each of these bundles is called a fasciculus (Latin = small bundle of twigs) and is surrounded by a layer of connective tissue called the perimysium. Each fasciculus consists of a number of muscle cells, and within the fasciculus, each individual muscle cell is surrounded by the endomysium, a fine sheath of delicate connective tissue.

The Anatomy of Exercise & Movement

Skeletal muscles come in a variety of shapes, due to the arrangement of their fasciculus (English = fascicles), depending on the function of the muscle in relation to its position and action. Parallel muscles have their fasciculus running parallel to the long axis of the muscle, e.g. sartorius. Pennate muscles have short fasciculus, which are attached obliquely to the tendon, and appear feather-shaped, e.g. rectus femoris. Convergent (triangular) muscles have a broad origin with the fasciculus converging toward a single tendon, e.g. pectoralis major. Circular (sphincter) muscles have their fasciculus arranged in concentric rings around an opening, e.g. orbicularis oculi.

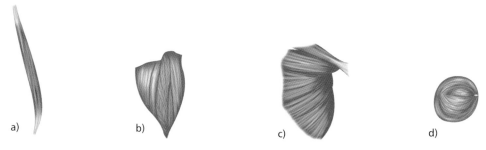

a)   b)   c)   d)

Figure 2.3: Muscle shapes: (a) parallel, (b) pennate, (c) convergent, and (d) circular.

Each muscle fiber is composed of small structures called muscle fibrils or myofibrils ('myo-' meaning 'muscle' in Latin). These myofibrils lie in parallel and give the muscle cell its striated appearance, because they are composed of regularly aligned myofilaments. Myofilaments are chains of protein molecules, which under microscope appear as alternate light and dark bands. The light isotropic (I) bands are composed of the protein actin. The dark anisotropic (A) bands are composed of the protein myosin. (A third protein called titin has been identified, which accounts for about 11% of the combined muscle protein content.) When a muscle contracts, the actin filaments move between the myosin filaments, forming cross-bridges, which results in the myofibrils shortening and thickening. (See 'The Physiology of Muscle Contraction'.)

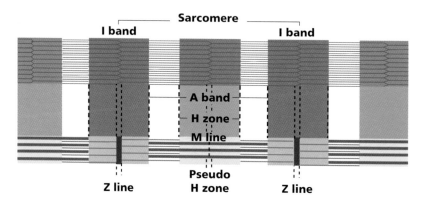

Figure 2.4: The myofilaments within a sarcomere. A sarcomere is bounded at both ends by the Z line; M line is the centre of the sarcomere; I band is composed of actin; A band is composed of myosin.

Commonly, the epimysium, perimysium, and endomysium extend beyond the fleshy part of the muscle, the belly, to form a thick ropelike tendon or broad, flat, sheet-like tendinous tissue, known as an aponeurosis. The tendon and aponeurosis form indirect attachments from muscles to the periosteum of bones or to the connective tissue of other muscles. However, more complex muscles may have multiple attachments, such as the quadriceps (four attachments). So typically a muscle spans a joint and is attached to bones by tendons at both ends. One of the bones remains relatively fixed or stable while the other end moves as a result of muscle contraction.

Each muscle fiber is innervated by a single motor nerve fiber, ending near the middle of the muscle fiber. A single motor nerve fiber and all the muscle fibers it supplies is known as a motor unit. The number of muscle fibers supplied by a single nerve fiber is dependent upon the movement required. When an exact, controlled degree of movement is required, such as in eye or finger movement, only a few muscle fibers are supplied; when a grosser movement is required, as in large muscles like gluteus maximus, several hundred fibers may be supplied.

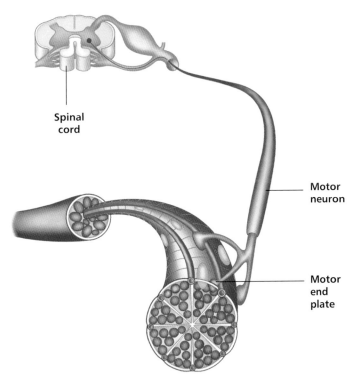

Spinal
cord

Motor
neuron

Motor
end
plate

Figure 2.5: A motor unit of a skeletal muscle.

Individual skeletal muscle fibers work on an 'all or nothing' principle, where stimulation of the fiber results in complete contraction of that fiber, or no contraction at all – a fiber cannot be 'slightly contracted'. The overall contraction of any named muscle involves the contraction of a proportion of its fibers at any one time, with others remaining relaxed.

The Physiology of Muscle Contraction

Nerve impulses cause the skeletal muscle fibers at which they terminate, to contract. The junction between a muscle fiber and the motor nerve is known as the neuromuscular junction, and this is where communication between the nerve and muscle takes place. A nerve impulse arrives at the nerve's endings, called synaptic terminals, close to the sarcolemma. These terminals contain thousands of vesicles filled with a neurotransmitter called acetylcholine (ACh). When a nerve impulse reaches the synaptic terminal, hundreds of these vesicles discharge their ACh. The ACh opens up channels, which allow sodium ions (Na+) to diffuse in. An inactive muscle fiber has a resting potential of about -95 mV. The influx of sodium ions reduces the charge, creating an end plate potential. If the end plate potential reaches the threshold voltage (approximately -50 mV), sodium ions flow in and an action potential is created within the fiber.

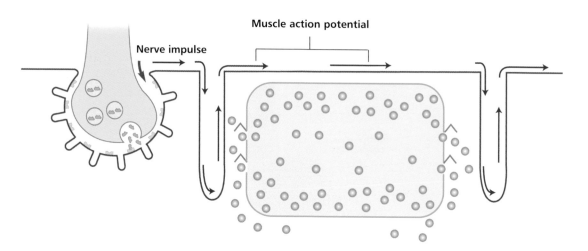

Figure 2.6: Nerve impulse triggering an action potential/muscle contraction.

No visible change occurs in the muscle fiber during (and immediately following) the action potential. This period, called the latent period, lasts from 3-10 msec. Before the latent period is over, the enzyme acetylcholinesterase breaks down the ACh in the neuromuscular junction, the sodium channels close, and the field is cleared for the arrival of another nerve impulse. The resting potential of the fiber is restored by an outflow of potassium ions. The brief period needed to restore the resting potential is called the refractory period.

So how does a muscle fiber shorten? This has been explained best by the sliding filament theory (Huxley & Hanson, 1954), which proposed that muscle fibers receive a nerve impulse (see above) that results in the release of calcium ions stored in the sarcoplasmic reticulum (SR). For muscles to work effectively, energy is required, and this is created by the breakdown of adenosine triphosphate (ATP). This energy allows the calcium ions to bind with the actin and myosin filaments to form a magnetic bond, which causes the fibers to shorten, resulting in the contraction. Muscle action continues until the calcium is depleted, at which point calcium is pumped back into the SR, where it is stored until another nerve impulse arrives.

Muscle Reflexes

Skeletal muscles contain specialized sensory units that are sensitive to muscle lengthening (stretching). These sensory units are called muscle spindles and Golgi tendon organs and they are important in detecting, responding to and modulating changes in the length of muscle.

Muscle spindles are made up of spiral threads called intrafusal fibers, and nerve endings, both encased within a connective tissue sheath, that monitor the speed at which a muscle is lengthening. If a muscle is lengthening at speed, signals from the intrafusal fibers will fire information via the spinal cord to the nervous system so that a nerve impulse is sent back, causing the lengthening muscle to contract. The signals give continuous information to/from the muscle about position and power (proprioception).

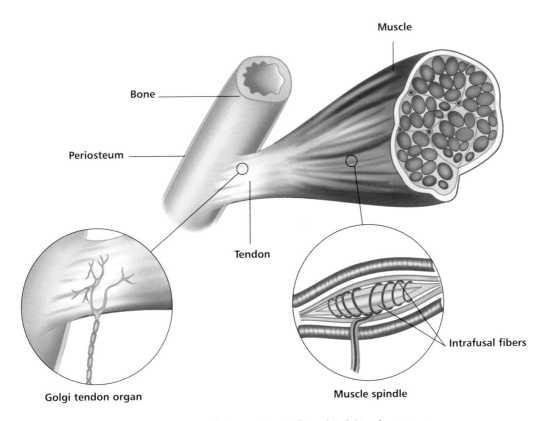

Figure 2.7: Anatomy of the muscle spindle and Golgi tendon organ.

Furthermore, when a muscle is lengthened and held, it will maintain a contractile response as long as the muscle remains stretched. This facility is known as the stretch reflex arc. Muscle spindles will remain stimulated as long as the stretch is held.

The classic clinical example of the stretch reflex is the knee jerk test, which involves activation of the stretch receptors in the tendon, which causes reflex contraction of the muscle attached, i.e. the quadriceps.

Whereas the muscle spindles monitor the length of a muscle, the Golgi tendon organs (GTO's) in the muscle tendon are so sensitive to tension in the muscle-tendon complex, that they can respond to the contraction of a single muscle fiber. The GTO's are inhibitory in nature, performing a protective function by reducing the risk of injury. When stimulated, the GTO's inhibit the contracting (agonist) muscles and excite the antagonist muscles.

Musculo-skeletal Mechanics

Most coordinated movement involves one attachment of a skeletal muscle remaining relatively stationary, whilst the attachment at the other end moves. The proximal, more fixed attachment is known as the origin, while the attachment that lies more distally, and moves, is known as the insertion. (However, attachment is now the preferred term for origin and insertion, as it acknowledges that muscles often work so that either end can be fixed whilst the other end moves.)

Most movements require the application of muscle force, which often is accomplished by agonists (or prime movers), which are primarily responsible for movement and provide most of the force required for movement; antagonists, which have to lengthen to allow for the movement produced by the prime movers, and play a protective role; and synergists (more specifically referred to as stabilizers, see page 21), which assist prime movers, and are sometimes involved in fine-tuning the direction of movement. A simple example is the flexion of the elbow, which requires shortening of the brachialis and biceps brachii (prime movers) and the relaxation of the triceps brachii (antagonist). The brachioradialis acts as the synergist by assisting the brachialis and biceps brachii.

Muscle movement can be broken down into three types of contractions: concentric, eccentric, and static (isometric). In many activities, such as running, Pilates and Yoga, all three types of contraction may occur to produce smooth, coordinated movement.

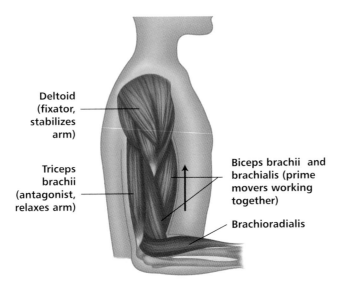

Deltoid (fixator, stabilizes arm)

Triceps brachii (antagonist, relaxes arm)

Biceps brachii and brachialis (prime movers working together)

Brachioradialis

Figure 2.8: Flexion of the elbow, where brachialis and biceps brachii act as the prime movers, triceps brachii as the antagonist, and brachioradialis as the synergist.

Skeletal muscles can be broadly classified into two types:

1. Stabilizers*, which essentially stabilize a joint. They are made up of slow-twitch fibers for endurance, and assist with postural holding. They can be further subdivided into primary stabilizers, which have very deep attachments, lying close to the axis of rotation of the joint; and secondary stabilizers, which are powerful muscles, with an ability to absorb large amounts of force. Stabilizers work against gravity, and tend to become weak and long over time (Norris, 1998). Examples include multifidus, transverse abdominus (primary), and gluteus maximus and adductor magnus (secondary).

2. Mobilizers* are responsible for movement. They tend to be more superficial although less powerful than stabilizers, but produce a wider range of motion. They tend to cross two joints, and are made of fast-twitch fibers that produce power but lack endurance. Mobilizers assist with rapid or ballistic movement and produce high force. With time and use, they tend to tighten and shorten. Examples include the hamstrings, piriformis and rhomboids.

A muscle's principle action, shortening, where the muscle attachments move closer together, is referred to as a concentric contraction. Because joint movement is produced, concentric contractions are also considered dynamic contractions. An example is that of holding an object, where the biceps brachii contracts concentrically, the elbow joint flexes and the hand moves up toward the shoulder.

Importantly, all skeletal muscles are stabilizers and mobilizers – it depends on the movement and position of the body as to how the muscles are reacting at the time.

A movement is considered to be an eccentric contraction where the muscle may exert force while lengthening. As with concentric contraction, because joint movement is produced, this is also referred to as a dynamic contraction. The actin filaments are pulled further from the centre of the sarcomere, effectively stretching it.

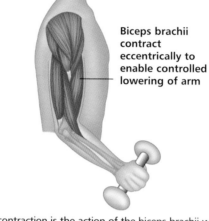

Biceps brachii contract eccentrically to enable controlled lowering of arm

Figure 2.9: An example of eccentric contraction is the action of the biceps brachii when the elbow is extended to lower a heavy weight. Here, biceps brachii is controlling the movement by gradually lengthening in order to resist gravity.

When a muscle acts without moving, force is generated but its length remains unchanged. This is known as static (isometric) contraction.

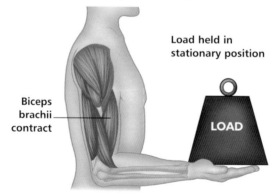

Load held in stationary position

Biceps brachii contract

LOAD

Figure 2.10: An example of static (isometric) contraction, where a heavy weight is held, with the elbow stationary and bent at 90 degrees.

Levers

A lever is a device for transmitting (but not creating force) and consists of a rigid bar moving about a fixed point (fulcrum). More specifically, a lever consists of an effort force, resistance force, rigid bar and a fulcrum. The bones, joints and muscles together form a system of levers in the body, where the joints act as the fulcrum, the muscles apply the effort and the bones carry the weight of the body part to be moved. Levers are classified according to the position of the fulcrum, resistance (load), and effort relative to each other.

In a first-class lever, the effort and resistance are located on opposite sides of the fulcrum. In a second-class lever, the effort and the resistance are located on the same side of the fulcrum, and the resistance is between the fulcrum and effort. Finally, in a third-class lever, the effort and resistance are located on the same side of the fulcrum, but the effort acts between the fulcrum and the resistance, and this is the most common type of lever in the human body.

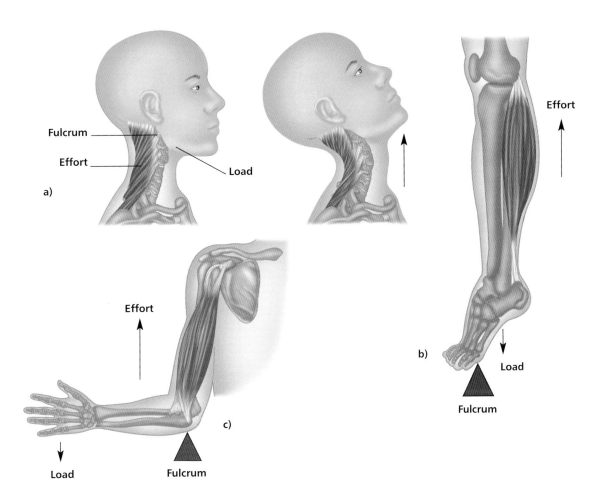

Figure 2.11: Examples of levers in the human body: (a) first-class lever, (b) second-class lever, and (c) third-class lever.

Generation of Force

The strength of skeletal muscle is reflected in its ability to generate force. If a weightlifter is able to lift 75kg, their muscles are capable of producing enough force to lift 75kg. Even when not trying to lift a weight, the muscles must still generate enough force to move the bones to which they are attached. A number of factors are involved in this ability to generate force, including the number and type of motor units activated, the size of the muscle and the angle of the joint.

Reciprocal Inhibition

Most movement involves the combined effort of two or more muscles, with one muscle acting as the prime mover. Most prime movers usually have a synergistic muscle to assist them. Furthermore, most skeletal muscles have one or more antagonists that performs the opposite action. A good example might be hip abduction, in which gluteus medius acts as the prime mover, with tensor fascia latae acting synergistically and the hip adductors acting as antagonists, being reciprocally inhibited by the action of the agonists.

Reciprocal inhibition (RI) is the physiological phenomenon in which there is an automatic inhibition of a muscle when its antagonist contracts. Under special circumstances both the agonist and antagonist can contract together, known as a co-contraction.

Muscles Involved in Breathing

Breathing is a vital part of life and sport, but plays a particularly important role in Pilates and Yoga, and it is worth noting the main skeletal muscles involved.

1.Diaphragm

The diaphragm is the main inspiratory muscle. Contraction of the muscle causes the dome of the diaphragm to descend, so enlarging the dimension of the thorax in all directions. The diaphragm contributes to spinal stability via an increase in intra-abdominal pressure, and with transversus abdominis, continually works to control trunk movement and enhance the breathing pattern during movement, particularly involving the extremities.

2. Intercostals

The outermost layer of the intercostal muscles is responsible for the lateral expansion of the chest and stabilization of the ribs during inspiration. Deep to them, the internal intercostals have an opposite action in forced expiration during exercise. The intercostals have a close anatomical connection with the internal and external oblique muscles.

3. Abdominal muscles

This is the main muscle group involved in forced expiration. These muscles alter the intra-abdominal pressure to assist the emptying of the lungs and transmit the pressure generated by the diaphragm. Intra-abdominal pressure is the pressure created within the trunk, in the closed cylinder of the diaphragm, pelvic floor and abdominal wall. Greater pressure adds stability to the trunk and pelvis.

4. Pelvic floor muscles

These are a collective group of muscles and soft tissue that makes up the base of the abdomino-pelvic cavity. These have a role in the maintenance of the intra-abdominal pressure and transference of the stability created by the respiratory process. Their main functions however are to support the internal pelvic organs and help to maintain continence.

5. Other muscle groups

Other muscle groups activated work with the main respiratory muscles but become activated when the exercise or asana becomes demanding, or when there is a change in position during the exercise or asana. They are needed to stabilize parts of the body to enhance the respiratory action.

The scalene muscles aid in deep inspiration by fixing the 1st and 2nd ribs, and maintain them during expiration against the contraction of the abdominal muscles. The sternocleidomastoid elevates the sternum and increases the forward and backward dimension of the chest during moderate to deep inspiration if the cervical spine is held stable. Serratus anterior assists in inspiration to laterally expand the rib cage, if the scapulae are stabilized.

The pectorals act in forced inspiration to raise the ribs, although the scapulae need to be stabilized by trapezius and serratus anterior to prevent scapular winging. Latissimus dorsi is involved in forced inspiration and expiration. Erector spinae helps in respiration by extending the thoracic spine and raising the rib cage. Quadratus lumborum stabilizes the 12th rib to prevent elevation during respiration.

Synovial Joints

Chapters 3–10 describe in detail the function of muscle groups and synovial joints in relation to movement. Joints, or articulations, have two functions: to hold bones together, and to give the rigid skeleton mobility. Immoveable (synarthrotic) and slightly moveable (amphiarthrotic) joints are found mainly in the axial skeleton, where joint stability is important to protect the internal organs. Synovial joints are freely moveable (diarthrotic), and so are found predominately in the limbs, where a greater range of movement is required; they have a number of distinguishing features: articular (hyaline) cartilage that covers the ends of the bones that form the joint; a joint cavity filled with lubricating synovial fluid, (a slippery fluid that provides a film that reduces friction); collateral or accessory ligaments that provide reinforcement and strength; bursae, fluid-filled sacs that provide cushioning; tendon sheaths that wrap themselves around tendons subject to friction, in order to protect them. Articular discs (menisci) are present in some synovial joints (e.g. knee), and act as shock absorbers. The six types of synovial joints are:

Plane or Gliding
Movement occurs when two, generally flat or slightly curved surfaces glide across one another. Examples: the acromioclavicular joint, and the sacro-iliac joint.

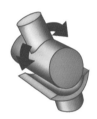

Hinge
Movement occurs around only one axis; a transverse one, as in the hinge of the lid of a box; the plane is sagittal. A protrusion of one bone fits into a concave or cylindrical articular surface of another, permitting flexion and extension. Examples: the interphalangeal joints, the elbow, and the knee.

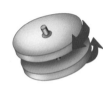

Pivot
Movement takes place around a vertical axis, like the hinge of a gate. A more or less cylindrical articular surface of bone protrudes into and rotates within a ring formed by bone or ligament. Example: the joint between the radius and the ulna at the elbow.

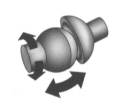

Ball-and-socket
Consists of a 'ball' formed by the spherical or hemispherical head of one bone that rotates within the concave 'socket' of another, allowing flexion, extension, adduction, abduction, circumduction, and rotation. Thus, they are multiaxial and allow the greatest range of movement of all joints. Examples: the shoulder and the hip joints.

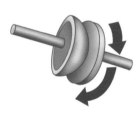

Condyloid
These have a spherical or ellipsoid articular surface that fits into a matching concavity. Permits flexion, extension, abduction, adduction, which combined together is called circumduction. Example: the wrist, the metacarpophalangeal joints of the fingers (but not the thumb).

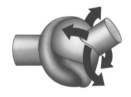

Saddle
Articulating surfaces have convex and concave areas, and so resemble two 'saddles' that join them together by accommodating each other's convex to concave surfaces. Allow even more movement than condyloid joints, for example, allowing the 'opposition' of the thumb to the fingers. Example: the carpometacarpal joint of the thumb.

Chapter

3

The Spine

The spine is the center of the body's universe, from a mechanical point of view. It is humanly impossible to move the body through space without the spine helping it to reach, bend over, turn around, stand up straight, or move the head to see.

The functions of the spine are **support**, **balance**, **connection**, **protection**, and **movement**. It supports and balances the erect posture. It connects the lower extremity to the upper extremity. The spine protects the spinal cord, which merges with the brain. Along with the articulating ribs, the spine protects the heart and lungs.

The Anatomy of Exercise & Movement

Actions (joint movements) occur in all three planes, moving the head and trunk. Joint actions are different from 'functions' (see page 27). The spine's joint actions are **flexion**, **extension**, **hyperextension**, **lateral flexion right and left**, and **rotation right and left**. Each part of the spine does some actions better than others.

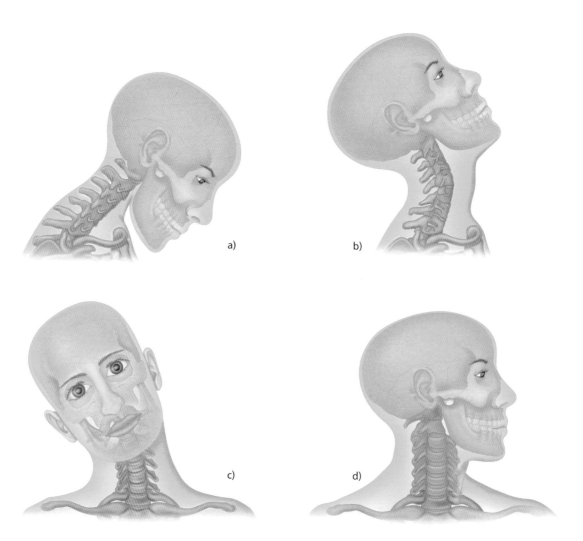

a)   b)

c)   d)

Figure 3.1: Neck movements; (a) flexion, (b) hyperextension, (c) lateral flexion, (d) rotation.

The Vertebral Spine

The vertebral spine is divided into the sections of **cervical**, **thoracic**, **lumbar**, **sacral**, and **coccyx**. They each have their own specialties.

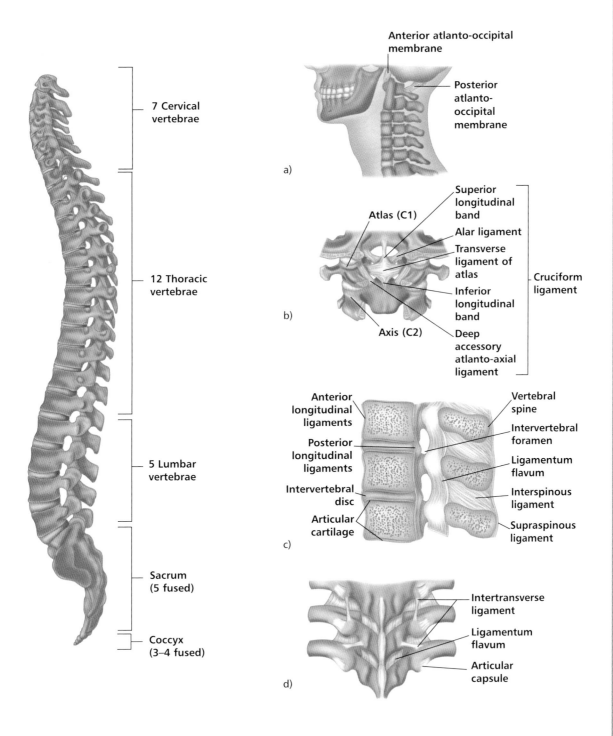

Figure 3.2: The vertebral spine; (a) atlanto-occipital joint, (b) atlanto-axial joint, (c) joints between vertebral bodies, and (d) joints between vertebral arches.

The main cervical area (C3-C7) is the most mobile, just slightly limited in side bending (lateral flexion). These vertebrae are small and thin, therefore easy to move.

C1 (the atlas) and C2 (the axis) are more specific. C1 articulates with the skull to create the **atlanto-occipital joint** (see figure 3.2a), where only flexion and extension can occur (the 'yes' motion). C1 and C2 join together to form the **atlanto-axial joint** (see figure 3.2b), where rotation occurs (the 'no' motion).

The 12 thoracic vertebrae can accomplish all spinal actions, but are restricted in hyperextension because of the posterior processes. This is the bony part of the spine that can be seen on the back; in the thoracic area they are long and mostly directed downward, limiting the 'backbend'. The 5 large, heavy lumbar vertebrae are limited in rotation, and the sacrum barely moveable after puberty. These naturally occurring limitations are caused by varying bone shapes that can lessen the range of motion.

The curves of these areas are necessary for balancing the weight of the head, thoracic cavity, sexual organs, and the pelvis (figure 3.2). This is an ingenious example of counterbalance against gravity.

Cervical Region

The cervical (neck) region, with its shallow anterior curve and 7 vertebrae, balances the head and allows it to turn and look at whatever, whoever, wherever. However, because it is the most moveable section, while balancing the skull's weight of 15 to 20 pounds, it must maintain constant equilibrium. Any deviation in load will affect not only the cervical area, but the rest of the spine as well.

Infants learn to balance the head as the spinal curves form. Remove support from the back of a young baby and the weight of the head and chest will topple it over. This is because muscles needed to provide the cervical, thoracic, and lumbar curves, which counteract each other, are still being developed. Once this power is established by kicking, crying, and throwing the arms about (crying, even wailing, develops deeper breathing muscles that aid the spine) the baby is able to hold its head up by the strength of the spinal muscles and ligaments acting on the curves. As growth continues, this delicate balancing act changes depending on how one sits, stands, walks, works, and sleeps. In this age of tension, the stress on the mechanical balance of the neck is eminent.

Stress affects this area through various means, especially by tightening shoulder and neck muscles. This can change posture, compress the vertebral discs, and misalign the spinal vertebrae. Active range of motion can alleviate the tightness and is the key to a healthy neck; a massage will help. This sounds so simple, when the area is extremely complex. Of the 24 articulating vertebrae and 31 pairs of spinal nerves, one small break in a particular area can paralyze the body for life.

Cervical Muscles

Most anterior neck muscles flex the cervical spine, bringing the head downward. When standing or sitting, gravity assists; the heavy weight of the head helps. This can cause weakness in the antagonist muscles, the extensors, if it becomes habitual. The strong pull of the large **sternocleidomastoid** muscle, along with small deeper muscles (**longus colli, longus capitis** and **rectus capitis anterior**) can pull the head down as well as support it.

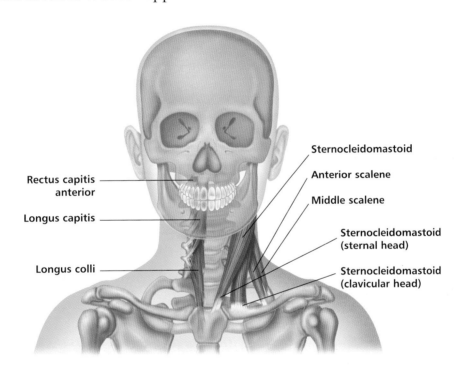

Figure 3.3: The anterior neck muscles.

The extensors on the back of the neck must concentrically contract to lift the head. Straightening the upper spine is work for many muscles: the **spleni, scalenes, upper erector spinae, semispinalis, deep posterior muscles,** and **obliquus capitis,** even the **trapezius.** These muscles also do either lateral flexion (along with the **levator scapula**) or rotation of the neck, so they are easy to strengthen because of the many actions they do. (The trapezius is addressed more specifically in Chapter 5.)

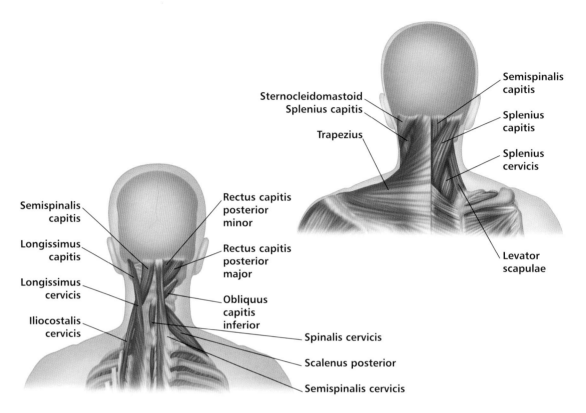

Figure 3.4: The posterior neck muscles.

Cervical Spine Stress

As a movement analyst, I have discovered that people overly engage in neck flexion, or bending the head forward. This is usually an unconscious movement, but a position that is often held for too long a time. Watch someone walking, and notice how much they look down. They are probably watching where they step, but after a time this becomes habit, particularly in the elderly. Others hang their head because the shoulders or back muscles are weak. Still others hide the chest and round the shoulders, bringing the head forward. Students sit and study, reading and writing with their heads down. In fact, anyone reading usually looks down to the text, not by moving their eyes, but by lowering the head. When sitting at the computer and looking at the monitor, where is the head? Most companies do not accommodate their employees by positioning the monitor at eye level; it is too high, too low, or too small, straining the neck and eyes. At home people do the same.

Bodies begin to compensate for various reasons; physical stress on the cervical and upper thoracic joints accumulates over time. This can lead to discomfort, pain, and/or disintegration of joints. If flexion is constant, the posterior portion of the spine will stretch while the anterior will compress. If the head is held too high, the opposite will happen.

Cervical Region Stretching and Range of Motion Exercises

Stretching can help achieve desired movement of the neck in all planes. This will also alleviate tense muscles.

The following level I exercises are recommended:

1. Using the floor as a strong base of support, lie on back with the head resting on the floor. Lengthen the cervical area by bringing the chin slightly closer to the throat. Allow weight of head to rest into the floor. Roll head to one side and let it hang, taking one full breath, then roll head to the other side without lifting it off the floor. Release the shoulders and relax on the exhale.

2. Sit or stand in front of a mirror. Close the eyes and center the head, then open the eyes and see where it really is. Using the mirror, attempt to center it directly between the shoulders, with both shoulders even. Begin to take the head through its full range of motion: flexion, extension, lateral flexion right and left, and rotation right and left. Do not allow the neck to hyperextend, or the shoulders to shift.

3. Use the left hand to take the head into lateral flexion left, while the right hand helps to hold the right shoulder down. Hold and use the exhale to relax; repeat on the other side.

To progress, try this.

4. *Advanced Inversions* (Level III)
   Find a position where the head can hang with gravity, not against it. This means inverting the body. Bending forward from a standing position (always slightly bend knees so the lumbar area is not over-stressed), hanging by the knees or ankles from a bar (not advised for everyone), or doing a handstand puts the head in this position. The cervical area will lengthen with gravity if it is free of head support.

Many people complain of neck weakness while doing a Pilates class. This is usually because the abdominal muscles are not yet strong enough to aid the pull of the trunk forward, and the front neck muscles have to work hard to hold the head up. As the abdominals increase in strength, the neck muscles can work more efficiently. The strong spine flexors (abdominals) are the focus of core exercises in Chapter 4.

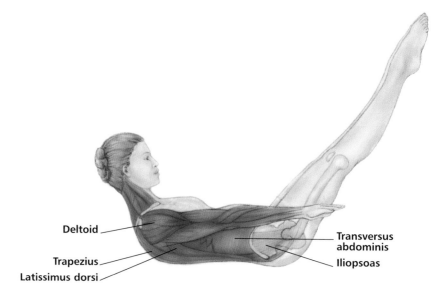

Deltoid

Trapezius

Latissimus dorsi

Transversus abdominis

Iliopsoas

Figure 3.5: The cervical position in Pilates 100.

TECHNIQUE

In Pilates floor work, from a supine position the head is brought up and forward (flexed) as the trunk also flexes. With gravity as the resisting force, abdominals that flex the thoracic and lumbar portions of the spine are strengthened, as well as the neck flexors.

With the head properly balanced on top of the cervical vertebrae and the neck strengthened, the next section of the spine can be addressed.

Thoracic Region

The 12 vertebrae make this the longest section of the spine, curving posteriorly (kyphosis). This curve accomplishes balance and support of the thoracic cavity. Imagine the articulation of the 12 thoracic vertebrae with the 12 ribs in the back, and the circumference of the ribs as they travel around the body to the front, connecting with the **sternum** (breastbone). Only the 2 lower ribs, the **floating ribs**, do not connect in front. The cavity created houses the heart and lungs.

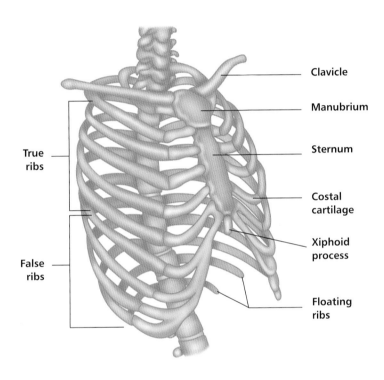

Figure 3.6: The thoracic cavity houses the heart and lungs.

The backward curve of the thoracic vertebrae is natural to most, but the following can pronounce it:

1. weak upper back muscles
2. tight chest muscles
3. the weight of the chest
4. fatigue
5. laziness

These conditions, added to by the pull of gravity, can advance the kyphosis, causing a person to appear slumped or rounded forward.

The Anatomy of Exercise & Movement

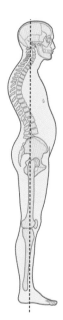

Figure 3.7: Kyphosis, a condition that causes a person to appear slumped or rounded forward.

Thoracic Muscles

The **erector spinae**, **semispinalis** and **deep posterior muscle groups** are the main workers of spinal extension, which is simply standing up straight.

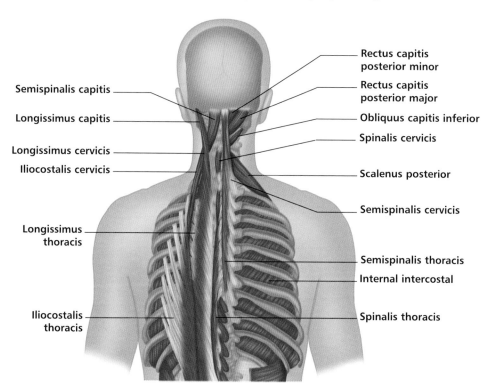

Semispinalis capitis

Longissimus capitis

Longissimus cervicis

Iliocostalis cervicis

Longissimus thoracis

Iliocostalis thoracis

Rectus capitis posterior minor

Rectus capitis posterior major

Obliquus capitis inferior

Spinalis cervicis

Scalenus posterior

Semispinalis cervicis

Semispinalis thoracis

Internal intercostal

Spinalis thoracis

Figure 3.8: Upper spine muscles.

Thoracic Region Stretching and Range of Motion Exercises

The best exercise regimens for an extended spine are Yoga and ballet. **People who practice Yoga have improved flexibility, balance, strength, circulation, posture and breathing.**

Yoga is possibly the most practiced discipline in the world, yet still rejected by many. This is usually due to the cultural or religious 'stigma' people relate to it. Throw those thoughts away; its lasting benefits are too important.

Muscles are responsible for the movement of bones. They do this best when they do not have to bear the burden of weight. Erect posture will allow them to do their job efficiently, without stress.

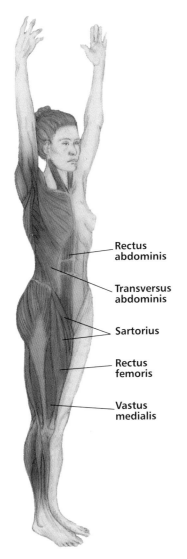

Rectus abdominis

Transversus abdominis

Sartorius

Rectus femoris

Vastus medialis

When a Yoga instructor explains the shoulder loop, or "bringing the shoulders back and down with the shoulder-blades sliding down the spine", the torso has lengthened. The **scapulae** are slightly adducted (closer to the spine), working the **trapezius** and **rhomboids**. This is also a main concept in Pilates, and useful in any form of exercise. The chest and ribs are open and relaxed, not 'pushing out', with the abdominals slightly in and lifted. In this position the spine can **breathe**, in a sense: the vertebrae are aligned one on top of the other with the discs un-compressed. Its curves are balanced, supple, and in symmetry with each other. Practice this postural work while sitting, standing, or walking, and feel the difference.

Figure 3.9: The supple, lengthened spine.

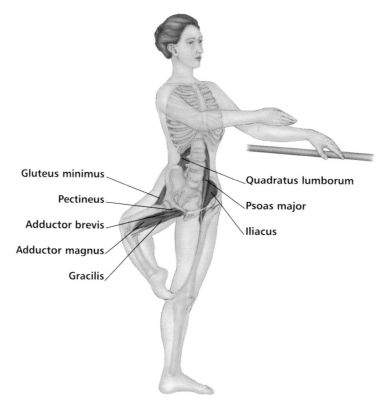

Gluteus minimus

Pectineus

Adductor brevis

Adductor magnus

Gracilis

Quadratus lumborum

Psoas major

Iliacus

Figure 3.10: Standing postures for balance, support, alignment for the ballet barre (level 1).

TECHNIQUE

Stand on one leg and take the other one to 'passé' position (bent knee, outward rotated hip, foot pointed to inside of standing knee). Keeping hips level, one can remain balanced while strengthening the legs and core. To increase strength, hold on to the barre or a wall and develop the supporting leg by doing pliés and relevés (bending the knee, then rising to the ball of the foot). Always track the knee over the toes.

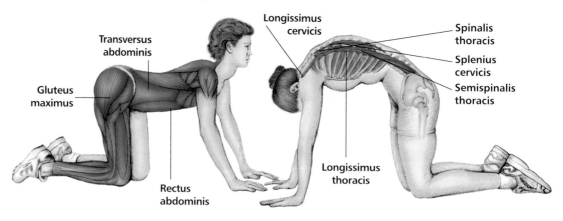

Transversus
abdominis

Gluteus
maximus

Rectus
abdominis

Longissimus
cervicis

Longissimus
thoracis

Spinalis
thoracis

Splenius
cervicis

Semispinalis
thoracis

Figure 3.11: Kneeling postures, for stretch and suppleness; (a) the "dog", (b) the "cat" (level 1).

The **dog**, or **cow** in Yoga: Begin on hands and knees, with wrists under shoulders and hips over knees. Arch (drop) the lumbar spine and allow the tailbone and head to lift slightly. Do this on an inhale, lifting the abdominals slightly for support and pulling shoulder-blades together.

The **cat**: Still on hands and knees, round the back into spinal flexion, dropping the coccyx and head. Exhale while pulling the abdominals up and separating the shoulder-blades.

Prone Postures for Flexibility and Strength

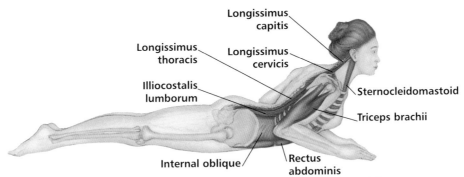

Figure 3.12: Bhujangasana (cobra pose), for the upper back (level I).

The **cobra** is an exercise for posterior upper back strength. Lying on the floor in a prone position, lift the upper body, keeping the head in line with the spine. Hands are under the shoulders with elbow along the sides of the ribs. Do not push into hands; allow the spine extensors to do the work. The pelvis should stay connected to the floor.

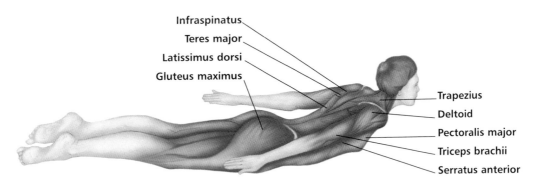

Figure 3.13: Salabhasana (locust pose), for the upper and lower back (level II).

The **locust** begins to strengthen the lower as well as upper spine muscles. When the legs are raised, it also strengthens the gluteus maximus and hamstrings. Reach the arms long by the sides as the upper and lower extremities lift off the floor. Do not hyperextend the neck.

The Anatomy of Exercise & Movement

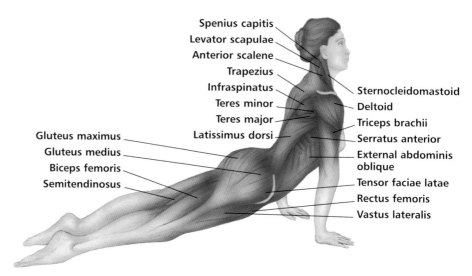

Spenius capitis
Levator scapulae
Anterior scalene
Trapezius
Infraspinatus
Teres minor
Teres major
Latissimus dorsi
Sternocleidomastoid
Deltoid
Triceps brachii
Serratus anterior
External abdominis oblique
Tensor faciae latae
Rectus femoris
Vastus lateralis
Gluteus maximus
Gluteus medius
Biceps femoris
Semitendinosus

Figure 3.14: Urdhva mukha svanasana (up dog) (level III).

TECHNIQUE

The **up dog** is a higher-level exercise because of stress on the arms and lower back. In prone position, the upper body hyperextends as the arms lengthen and hands are pressed into the floor. If abdominals are engaged, the pelvis can lift off the floor. The feet are extended. Looking straight forward will reduce stress on the cervical area.

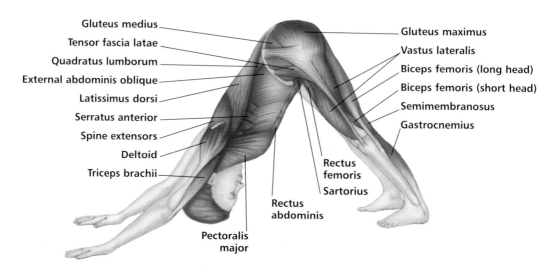

Gluteus medius
Tensor fascia latae
Quadratus lumborum
External abdominis oblique
Latissimus dorsi
Serratus anterior
Spine extensors
Deltoid
Triceps brachii
Gluteus maximus
Vastus lateralis
Biceps femoris (long head)
Biceps femoris (short head)
Semimembranosus
Gastrocnemius
Rectus femoris
Sartorius
Rectus abdominis
Pectoralis major

Figure 3.15: Adho mukha svanasana (down dog), depending on the position (levels I–III).

TECHNIQUE

The **down dog** is one of the most efficient exercises in Yoga. It lengthens the spine, hamstrings, and calves, engages the core, and strengthens shoulder muscles. In prone position, begin on hands and knees.
Level I: Tuck the toes under, keep tailbone lifted and reach arms forward on the floor, spreading fingers.
Level II: Lift knees off floor but keep them bent while pushing body weight back toward the legs. Let the head hang between the arms.
Level II–III: Assume level II position. Straighten knees, reach tailbone high while pushing weight out of the arms toward the thighs. Keep shoulders away from ears by pulling blades down while the shoulder joint outward rotates. Let the head hang free. Feel the foundation of both hands and feet and engage the core (pictured).

Supine Postures for Flexibility and Strength

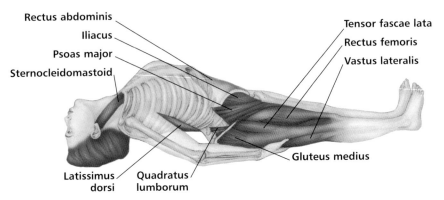

Figure 3.16: Matsyasana (fish pose) (level II shown). For level III, raise arms to ceiling.

TECHNIQUE

In supine position, extend the body and place hands under tailbone with arms long. Lift the sternum and allow the thoracic spine to hyperextend from the floor. The head is balanced on the floor, as well as the tailbone. Using a blanket, block, or bolster horizontally under T4-7 will aid the posture. Some people might also need a blanket or support under the head or knees. Fish opens the chest and strengthens the back.

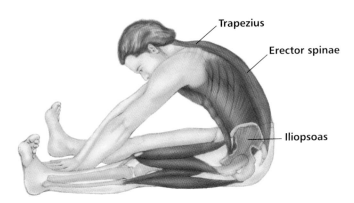

Figure 3.17: Pilates spine stretch (level I).

TECHNIQUE

The Pilates **spine stretch** is done in a small straddle position, feet flexed. Begin by sitting against a wall with the spine straight and arms reaching forward. As the spine rounds forward (flexion), pull the abdominals toward the wall; the lower back should not leave the wall. Roll back up the wall through each vertebra to straighten.

In the weight room, **good mornings** work the spine in constant contraction of the extensor muscles.

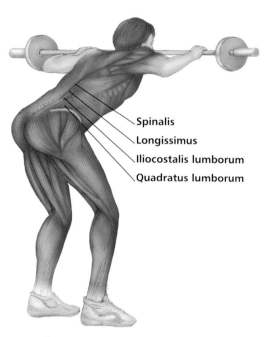

- Spinalis
- Longissimus
- Iliocostalis lumborum
- Quadratus lumborum

Figure 3.18: Good mornings.

Using a slow, controlled, full range of movement, lower the torso toward the ground by bending at the waist, keeping the back straight with the hips and knees slightly flexed. Return by raising the torso until the trunk is over the legs. Inhale on the up phase. This exercise can be repeated 8–12 times in 2–3 sets.

A second exercise, **deadlifts**, is a popular exercise for body builders, sometimes done in preparation for power lifting. Even though the main action in a deadlift squat is hip and knee extension against gravity and weight, a secondary movement is also spine extension; some of these muscles are pictured below.

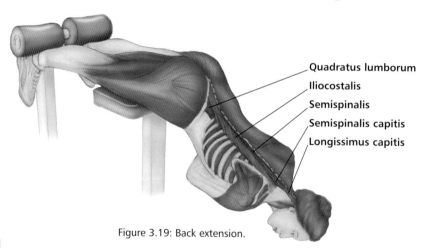

- Quadratus lumborum
- Iliocostalis
- Semispinalis
- Semispinalis capitis
- Longissimus capitis

Figure 3.19: Back extension.

Place body in position shown, allowing hip joints to flex over bench. Torso can begin in low, stretched position; the strength of the exercise is raising the torso to hyperextend the spine against resistance. This exercise is considered level II or III depending on the condition of the lower spine. If lumbar discs are aggravated, do not perform this exercise.

Flexibility Exercises

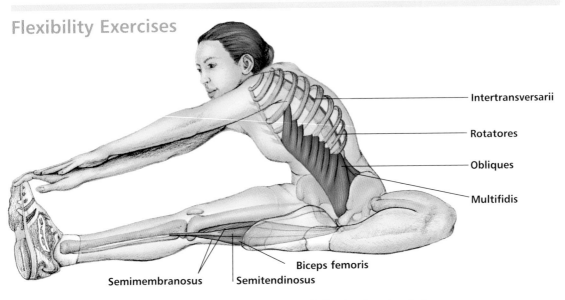

Intertransversarii

Rotatores

Obliques

Multifidis

Biceps femoris

Semimembranosus   Semitendinosus

Figure 3.20: Sitting side reach stretch (for the thoracic spine).

TECHNIQUE

Sit with one leg straight out to the side and the toes pointing up. Bring the other foot up to the knee and let the head extend forward. Reach toward the outside of the toes with both hands, keeping the shoulders down away from the ears. Bend knee if the hamstrings are too tight.

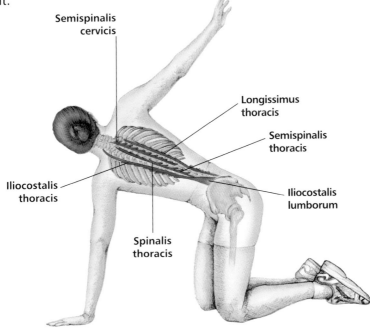

Semispinalis
cervicis

Longissimus
thoracis

Semispinalis
thoracis

Iliocostalis
thoracis

Iliocostalis
lumborum

Spinalis
thoracis

Figure 3.21: Kneeling back rotation stretch (for the thoracic spine).

TECHNIQUE

Kneel on the ground in table position and raise one arm. Then rotate shoulders and middle back while looking upward. Use a blanket under knees for support if needed. Spinal twists are excellent for stretching and strengthening the spine, as well as releasing toxins and stress. There are many spinal twists that can be done either standing, sitting, kneeling, or lying supine.

The Anatomy of Exercise & Movement

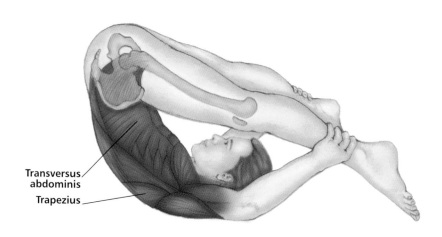

Transversus
abdominis

Trapezius

Figure 3.22: Pilates open leg rocker for the full spine (level III).

TECHNIQUE

Begin this position sitting in the Pilates **Table** or **Teaser**, balancing just behind the tailbone. Use a blanket under the sit bones and spine if needed. The object is to roll back on the spine articulating through each vertebra; do not roll onto the neck, only the lower to mid spine. If this does not feel good on the spine, do not do it, just work on the sitting balance if it does not bother the lower spine.

This exercise is done slowly, only 3–4 repetitions, coming up to sitting in balance between each roll. This also becomes a great exercise for the abdominals and psoas (see Chapter 4).

Level II – knees bent
Level III – knees straight

The opposite movement of extension in the sagittal plane is flexion. In the thoracic area, it is accomplished by contraction of the abdominals. This, along with the lumbar/sacral areas of the spine, is addressed in Chapter 4.

Myths of the Upper Spine Dispelled

Common patterns of neck position can lead to dysfunction

Typically the neck is in constant overuse: holding the head up against gravity, or turning it in some way. Even in rest, the neck is compromised if one lies on the stomach. Movement patterns learned are hard to break, and people tend to allow the neck, the most mobile area of the spine, to take the brunt of body positions. **The cervical vertebrae need to rest in neutral position. Lying on the back with the head aligned with the spine is the best sleeping position.**

Using the arms extensively can weaken the upper spine

Use of the arms can strengthen the areas related to them, specifically the cervical and thoracic spinal areas. However, extensive use (lifting, reaching, throwing, swimming for long periods of time) can tire the same areas, so the stabilizing muscles need to be properly engaged. There are specific exercises that can address this. **The best stabilizing exercises for the spine are found in Yoga positions such as the down dog, where correct placement of the shoulder joint and girdle properly align and engage the neck and thoracic muscles as they lengthen.**

Connective tissue is a culprit in mobility

Injury, range of motion, tension, and positioning can affect the connective tissue between the vertebrae, sometimes leading to dysfunction, pain, even degeneration over time. The small connective tissue may become inflamed, displaced, or torn. Scar tissue can be a result, leading to chronic stiffness. The condition is hard to diagnose and treat, but not impossible. **Manual therapy can help alleviate connective tissue problems, as well as use of positive imagery and correct exercise.**

Main Muscles Involved in Movements of the Spine

Atlanto-occipital & Atlanto-axial Joints

Flexion
Longus Capitis; Rectus Capitis Anterior;
Sternocleidomastoideus (anterior fibers)

Extension
Semispinalis Capitis; Splenius Capitis; Rectus
Capitis Posterior Major; Rectus Capitis
Posterior Minor; Obliquus Capitis Superior;
Longissimus Capitis; Trapezius;
Sternocleidomastoideus (posterior fibers)

Rotation and Lateral Flexion
Sternocleidomastoideus; Obliquus Capitis
Inferior; Obliquus Capitis Superior; Rectus
Capitis Lateralis; Longissimus Capitis;
Splenius Capitis

Intervertebral Joints (Cervical Region)

Flexion
Longus Colli; Longus Capitis;
Sternocleidomastoideus

Extension
Longissimus Cervicis; Longissimus Capitis;
Splenius Capitis; Splenius Cervicis;
Semispinalis Cervicis; Semispinalis Capitis;
Trapezius; Interspinales; Iliocostalis Cervicis

Rotation and Lateral Flexion
Longissimus Cervicis; Longissimus Capitis;
Splenius Capitis; Splenius Cervicis;
Multifids; Longus Colli; Scalenus Anterior;
Scalenus Medius; Scalenus Posterior;
Sternocleidomastoideus; Levator Scapulae;
Iliocostalis Cervicis; Intertransversarii

Intervertebral Joints (Thoracic & Lumbar Regions)

Flexion
Muscles of Anterior Abdominal Wall

Extension
Erector Spinae; Quadratus Lumborum;
Longus Colli; Interspinalis; Intertransversarii;
Multifidis; Rotatores; Semispinalis Thoracis

Rotation and Lateral Flexion
Iliocostalis Lumborum; Iliocostalis Thoracis;
Multifidis; Rotatores; Intertransversarii;
Quadratus Lumborum; Muscles of Anterior
Abdominal Wall

Chapter

4 The Core

The body's **core** gets much attention, but what is it, really? Depending on the source, it can be anything from the abdominals, to the complete torso. For this text, it will be clarified as the area from the lumbar spine to the pelvis, generally thought of as the central core. Both lower spine and the pelvis are interdependent; they must be in balance and alignment with each other to function properly. Any incongruence will affect other areas, from the upper spine to the feet; essentially the entire length of the body.

Lumbar Region

There are five lumbar vertebrae, approximately located in the center of the body. They are larger, thicker, and therefore heavier than the other bones of the spine. They have a lordotic curve, meaning anterior, or toward the front, which counterbalances the thoracic posterior curve. The discs (the cartilage in between the bones) are one-third the thickness of the vertebral bodies, which allows for increased mobility in flexion, extension, and lateral bending. Rotation is limited due to the straight projection, short length, and bulky properties of the posterior spinal processes, along with the orientation of the facets (articulating surfaces of a vertebra process).

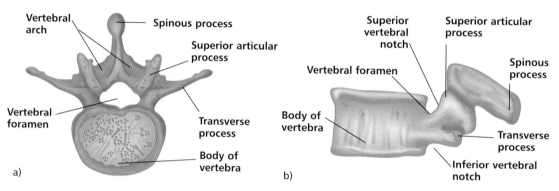

Figure 4.1: Lumbar vertebrae (L3); a) superior view, b) lateral view.

Lumbar Muscles

The **abdominals** are the main muscle group that flexes the lumbar and thoracic spine. This is the action where the torso bends forward, or curls into the fetal position. If one does this against resistance, such as gravity, the muscles strengthen. Each of the four abdominal muscles will be addressed separately, but as a unit because of their location and attachment to the anterior portion of the spine, they are mostly responsible for the health of the lower back.

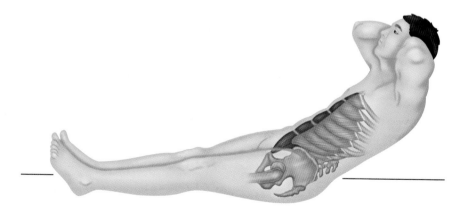

Figure 4.2: Curl up, supine position.

Abdominal Muscle #1: Rectus Abdominis

This muscle is the most superficial (closest to the skin) and longest of the abdominals, so therefore the one that is "seen" the most. Its fibers run vertically and are striated in the upper portion, producing that infamous 6-pack look. It is actually just a segmented appearance in the muscle fibers, seen mostly if a person is very lean.

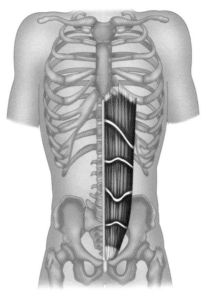

Figure 4.3: The rectus abdominis.

To strengthen the rectus abdominis, perform exercises that will **flex the spine** against resistance, and perform them correctly. Lie on the back and roll up, as in a sit-up, and the spine has flexed, with gravity as the resistance. Working against resistance is the most important aspect; when bending forward from a standing or sitting position, the spine is flexing, but gravity is helping, not resisting, so the abdominal muscles are not in a contracted, strong-enough state to increase strength.

If the rectus abdominis is engaged in the correct manner, it can support the lower back, and help stabilize the pelvis by lifting it (this is one of the core concepts of the Pilates method, and therefore why it works). To *engage* a muscle means to work it; to work it means it contracts. **Muscle contraction** is the force, or work, that a muscle does to produce joint movement. The muscle belly can shorten (**concentric contraction**), lengthen (**eccentric contraction**), or stay the same length (**isometric contraction**). A muscle cannot flex, it can only contract (a joint flexes – beware of muscle 'myths'!). Also, **a muscle must *cross* a joint to move it**. The rectus abdominis contracts to produce flexion of the spine because its fibers wrap around with the sheaths of the other abdominals laterally to posteriorly, therefore aiding the thoracic and lumbar areas. Its main attachments anteriorly are on ribs 5 through 7 as well as the xyphoid process at the end of the sternum, and the pubis symphysis. These attachment points are brought closer together when the muscle concentrically contracts.

Most muscles can do more than one action at a given joint. The rectus abdominis can laterally flex the spine (bend the trunk to the side) as well as flex it forward. It does lateral flexion **ipsilaterally** (the right rectus abdominis bends the spine to the right; the left rectus abdominis does the same to the left). It also assists the other three abdominals in compression of the abdominal area, which prevents hyperextension of the lumbar area (a 'sway' back is excessive hyperextension).

In a sit-up, the rectus abdominis concentrically contracts (shortens) to bring the trunk off the floor. Once the trunk is high enough and the hips become involved, the strong hip flexors can help, or sometimes take over. Therefore, the most effective part of the sit-up for the abdominal area is the first half of the sit-up, when the abdominals tend to be more isolated and gravity is most effective.

When rolling back down, the rectus abdominis eccentrically contracts (lengthens). The muscle is still contracting against resistance (gravity) to keep the back from slamming into the floor. Therefore, the rectus abdominis is the main mover during the full phase of a sit-up (see figure 4.2). In figure 4.4 below, flexion of the spine is clearly shown, although the flexor muscles do not work hard here, since gravity is helping. It is more a stretch for the posterior muscles.

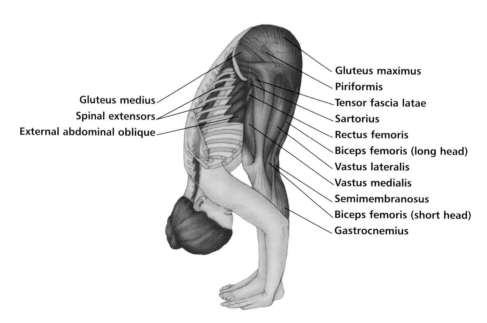

Figure 4.4: Flexion of spine during uttanasana (standing forward bend).

Rectus Abdominis Strengthening Exercises

1. *Side-bending* (Level I)

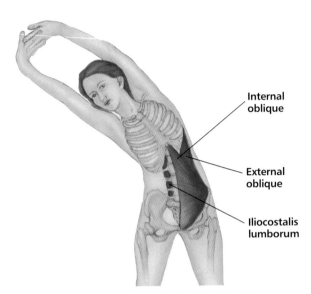

Figure 4.5: Side-bending (level I).

Stand with feet shoulder-width apart. Keep body upright and bend to the left or to the right. Can be performed sitting, kneeling, or standing, and is both a strength and stretch exercise for the abdominals. Arms overhead will add difficulty.

2. *The Partial Sit-up* (Levels I–II)

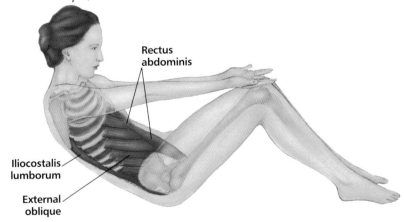

Figure 4.6: The partial sit-up (levels I–III).

Lie on back (supine position) with knees bent, and feet on the floor. Flex the spine (always exhale when flexing) coming up halfway, and roll back down through each vertebrae on the "inhale".

The Anatomy of Exercise & Movement

3. *The Pilates 100* (Level II)

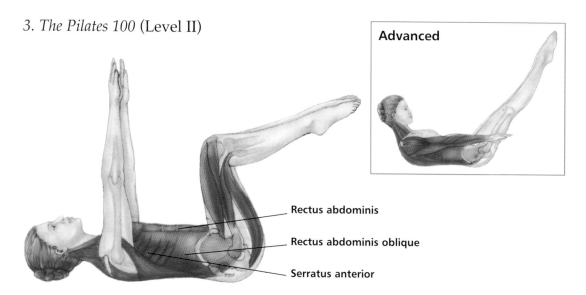

Advanced

Rectus abdominis

Rectus abdominis oblique

Serratus anterior

Figure 4.7: The Pilates 100 (level II).

TECHNIQUE

Lie on back, then flex the spine with the feet either on or off the floor, knees bent (legs straight and/or lowered is more advanced); the position is held, and the '100' is how many times the arms pump (arms are held straight in at the sides of the body). This position also strengthens the anterior neck muscles.

4. *Leg Lowers (as opposed to lifts)* (Levels II–III)

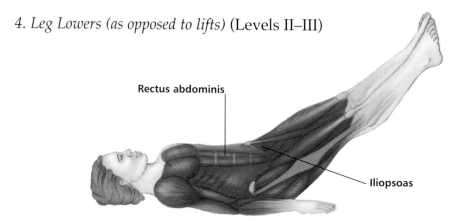

Rectus abdominis

Iliopsoas

Figure 4.8: Leg lowers (levels II–III).

TECHNIQUE

Level II: Lie on back, legs raised with knees slightly bent. Hands can be underneath tailbone (easier) or at sides/off the floor (more difficult). Lower legs to 45 degrees while pressing abdominals toward spine, then raise legs with knees bent; try to lift hips off floor slightly at the end of the leg lift.

Level III: Keep legs straight throughout entire exercise. The head can be lifted, as in the advanced inset above.

Repetition of the movement until fatigue is one of the best ways to overload the muscles being worked. **Strength is increased by overloading**. In Yoga, postures are held (isometric contraction) to create overload. In Pilates and weight training, movement is repeated using concentric and eccentric contraction.

The speed of the repetitions is an individual choice, but be reminded that **slower** may actually be more beneficial; taking time to connect the mind with the body, working the correct muscles the right way and slowly, can exhaust the targeted muscles. When the last movement is completed, it should be at a point of fatigue.

Seven points to keep in mind, for any age and level:

1. **Any exercise that flexes the spine against resistance** (gravity, weights, etc.), or laterally flexes the spine, will contract (work) the rectus abdominis.

2. A muscle needs to overload to increase strength – **repetitions and sets** are one of the best ways to do this, completing at least 8 repetitions in 2–3 sets, with fatigue the indicator of overload. (In Pilates, the emphasis is on slower and less repetitions, which can also tire the muscle.) Weight can be added to increase overload.

3. **There is a right and left side to every muscle** – work both sides equally.

4. **Have strength and length as the goal** – the desired appearance will happen eventually.

5. **The 6-pack is defined by three tendinous intersections** that the rectus fibers adhere to, which are visible as 'grooves' when the muscle contracts. If this look is desired, body fat must be on the lean side, and the muscle will most likely have to be 'engaged' to be seen.

6. **BREATHE!** This is actually an exercise for all four abdominals.

7. **ENJOY!**

Abdominal Muscle #2: External Obliques

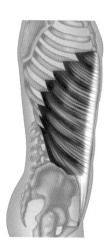

This muscle lies under the rectus abdominis, not directly, but more lateral to it. When both left and right sides of the muscle contract together, it assists the rectus in flexion of the spine. When one side contracts, it helps in lateral flexion (the right external oblique bends the spine to the right side, defined previously as ipsilateral). It is primarily a rotator of the spine **contra-laterally** (the right external oblique rotates the spine to the left, or opposite side).

Figure 4.9: The external obliques.

External Obliques Strengthening Exercises

1. Windmills (Level I)

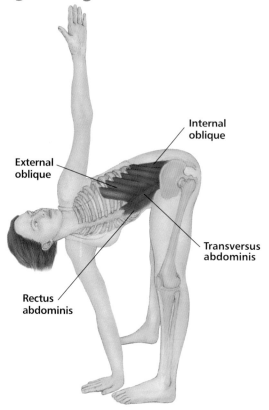

Figure 4.10 Windmills (level I).

TECHNIQUE

Standing with arms out to sides, touch right hand to left ankle, stand up and repeat to other side. This will do all three actions of the external oblique, and provide both a strength and stretch exercise. It is mild because rotation is minimal against resistance – bend knees slightly to keep from hyperextending them.

2. *The Pilates Saw* (Level I–II)

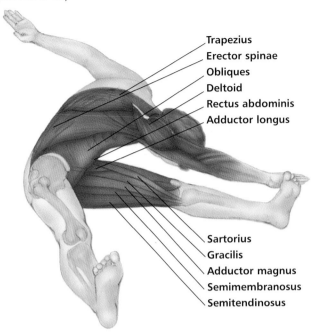

Trapezius
Erector spinae
Obliques
Deltoid
Rectus abdominis
Adductor longus

Sartorius
Gracilis
Adductor magnus
Semimembranosus
Semitendinosus

Figure 4.11: The Pilates saw.

TECHNIQUE

Sitting straight with legs straddled about two feet apart, arms out to sides: rotate to the right, then bend forward, reaching the left hand toward the right foot. Exhale and deepen the stretch of the spine by pulling the abdominals against the spine. Return by rolling through spine to upright position and repeat on the opposite side.

3. *Twisting Sit-ups/Pilates Criss-cross* (Level II)

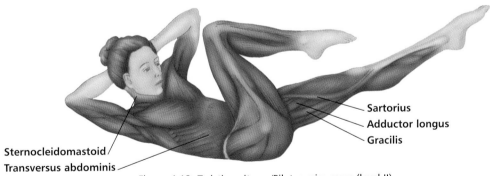

Sartorius
Adductor longus
Gracilis

Sternocleidomastoid
Transversus abdominis

Figure 4.12: Twisting sit-ups/Pilates criss-cross (level II).

TECHNIQUE

Lie on back, hands behind head without pulling on neck, elbows open; knees bent, feet on or off floor. Lift back a few inches off the floor, eyes to ceiling or abdominals. Move right elbow toward left knee, return to center, and repeat to the other side. Inhale on the twist, making sure the spine rotates as much as possible while hips remain stable; exhale in the center (always press abdominals toward spine while exhaling). This technique is ideal for all abdominals, especially the obliques.

4. Roman Chair Rotational Crunches (Levels I–III)

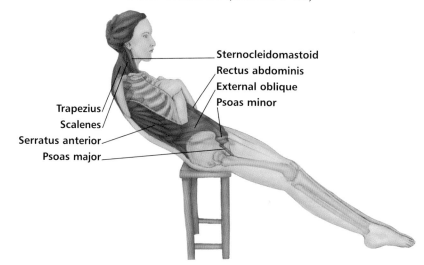

Sternocleidomastoid
Rectus abdominis
External oblique
Psoas minor
Trapezius
Scalenes
Serratus anterior
Psoas major

Figure 4.13: Roman chair rotational crunches (levels I–III).

TECHNIQUE

(This exercise is very hard on the lumbar (lower) spine, so make sure that the abdominals are strong to begin with.) Sit sideways on a bench with feet stabilized on the floor. Lie back slowly in a curled (flexed) position until parallel with the floor; return. To isolate the obliques, rotate the spine, alternating sides on the return.

Abdominal Muscle #3: Internal Obliques

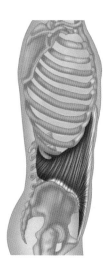

Lying under the external oblique and at right angles to it, the internal oblique also aids in flexion of the spine, lateral flexion, and is a primary rotator. When both sides contract (bilateral contraction), flexion happens; when one side contracts (unilateral), the resulting actions are lateral flexion and rotation. The internal oblique rotates to the same side (right internal oblique rotates and laterally flexes the spine to the right) working ipsilaterally. (The external oblique rotates to the opposite side, or contralaterally, as explained on page 54.)

Figure 4.14: The internal obliques.

The same exercises listed for the external obliques will also work the internal obliques.

Abdominal Muscle #4: Transversus Abdominis

The transversus abdominis is the deepest abdominal muscle. Its muscle fibers run horizontally around the waist, hence the term "the waist cincher", or girdle. It attaches posteriorly (toward the back) to the thoraco-lumbar fascia, but does not work the spine in the usual sense. It actually reduces the diameter of the abdomen, or 'pulls the belly in'. This muscle can be felt when placing hands on the sides of the waist and coughing.

The transversus abdominis also attaches to the inguinal ligament (running from the anterior superior iliac spine to the pubic tubercle) and the iliac crest, both parts of the pelvic girdle. **This makes the transversus abdominis an extremely important muscle, due to the fact that it is a stabilizer of both the spine and the pelvis.**

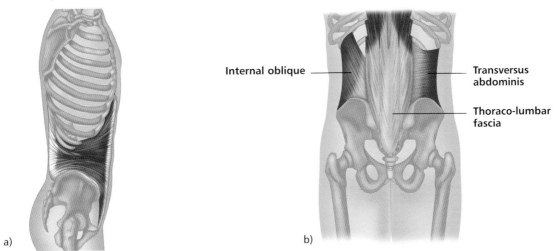

Internal oblique

Transversus abdominis

Thoraco-lumbar fascia

a)

b)

Figure 4.15: a) The transversus abdominis,
b) transversus abdominis and internal obliques inserting into thoraco-lumbar fascia.

Transversus Abdominis Exercises

The best exercises for the transversus abdominis are ones that involve deep breathing. This muscle concentrically contracts when exhaling. Forced expiration in any type of breathing exercise will activate the transversus abdominis. Certain types of Yogic breathing, called **pranayamas**, are good examples. It can also be activated in any exercise, such as sit-ups and push-ups, by exhaling deeply when moving against gravity / resistance. A good stretch for transversus abdominis would be the **rising stomach stretch**.

The Anatomy of Exercise & Movement

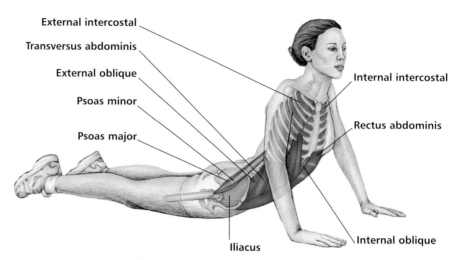

Figure 4.16. Rising stomach stretch.

TECHNIQUE

Lie face down and bring the hands close to the shoulders. Keep the hips on the ground, look forward and rise up by straightening the arms.

The "Weave"

The abdominals are located one on top of the other and in this pattern they look woven, not unlike the fabric in a piece of cloth: fibers are woven together to provide strength in the material. The abdominals are layered, and the muscle fibers also cross each other at angles to provide strength.

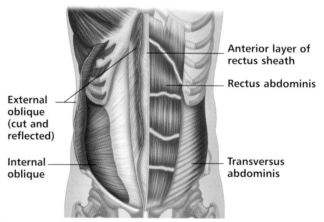

Figure 4.17: The 'weave'; all four abdominal muscles together.

If each abdominal muscle is exercised *properly*, the core area will become stronger and more supportive of the lower back and pelvis. Emphasize: **PROPERLY**. Some conventional exercise routines tend to build muscle bulk; in the case of the abdominals, flat seems more desirable than bulk. Some of the best exercises for abdominal strength and 'length', producing a flatter appearance, are included in conditioning techniques such as the Pilates method. Pilates has been labeled 'trendy', yet dancers and athletes have studied it for years. Joseph Pilates developed the system in the 1920s, and it has become an excellent training, conditioning, and rehabilitation system used throughout the world. I believe it is currently more popular because other workout methods have fallen short of what people really want and need.

The *look* of the abdominals is secondary; whether flat or round, the all-important thing is strength. People that have the flattest stomachs because they are thin can sometimes have the weakest ones. This can lead to lower back pain or incorrect posture. So, just because someone is thin, does *not* mean they don't have to exercise. On the other hand, possibly overweight or 'out-of-shape' people need the correct exercises and the patience to understand how the body has to work to achieve results. It is surprising that so much attention is brought to the look, when many people are not happy with how they look no matter what, and would just feel better if they were stronger and more well-balanced.

Abdominal strength increases the chances of surviving lower back problems. In the United States alone this condition has become a 'disease' of unknown proportions causing an infinite number of insurance claims, unemployment, and disability, resulting in a loss of billions of dollars. There are other causes, of course, but if the abdominals are strong, most times the debilitating pain of back injury can be avoided.

Use all four abdominals, they are meant to work together. Allow them to come in on the exhale, and out on the inhale. Lengthen without overworking the center. Relax the shoulders and breathe through the rib cage.

Stretching
While the benefits of stretching are debatable, most researchers agree that stretching a muscle carefully will increase range of motion (ROM) over time, allowing for better and safer joint mobility. Stretching can be done before, during, or after exercise, and is very effective following a particularly hard workout when the muscles have concentrically contracted (shortened, or bulked). Once the muscles begin to relax, stretching can be done. **A tense muscle cannot stretch.** Lengthen by stretching the muscle while it is relaxed, then hold for two seconds or more. If the stretch reflex has not been activated, the position can be held longer.

The **stretch reflex** is a function of the neuromuscular system (see Chapter 2, page 20). It is a reflexive contraction of the muscle being stretched, a built-in protective mechanism that helps prevent over-mobility of a joint. In other words, when the muscle is stretched too far, it will *tell* you to stop the stretch before it is injured. If one is careful while stretching and *listens* to the muscle, a stretch can be held comfortably. Hold far and long enough to feel what is stretching, but no further unless it is not painful. Breathe throughout the stretch, and relax.

The abdominals can be stretched just like any other muscle. Stretching will lead to better mobility of the spine.

The Anatomy of Exercise & Movement

Abdominal Stretching Exercises

1. *The Half-bridge* (Level I)

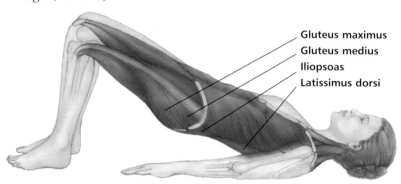

Gluteus maximus
Gluteus medius
Iliopsoas
Latissimus dorsi

Figure 4.18: The half-bridge (level I).

TECHNIQUE

Lying on back with knees bent and feet flat on floor, curl the tailbone off the floor; begin to raise hips as high as what feels comfortable. Weight should be evenly distributed to both feet and shoulder-blades.

2. *Spinal Twists* (Level I)

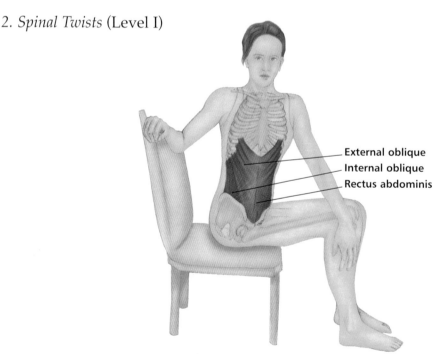

External oblique
Internal oblique
Rectus abdominis

Figure 4.19: Spinal twists (level I).

TECHNIQUE

Level I (beginning): Sitting on a chair, feet on floor; place right hand on the back of the chair, left hand on right knee; rotate spine to the right, beginning with lower back first, then mid, then upper back and neck. Spine must be extended (straight). Repeat on the other side. Do not over-twist the lumbar spine; it can lead to injury as rotation is not its best action.

3. *Spinal Twists* (Levels II–III)

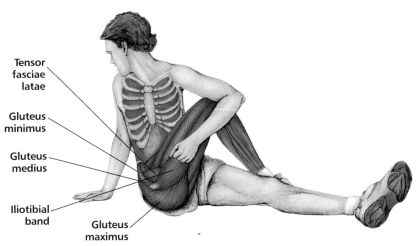

Figure 4.20: Spinal twists (levels II–III).

Level II: Sit on floor with left leg extended, right leg bent with thigh against chest, spine extended. Right foot can be on inside or outside of left knee. Hold right knee with left forearm, place right hand behind right hip on floor; rotate the spine to the right. Repeat on the other side.

Level III (advanced): Follow previous level II exercise, except bend left leg underneath right, and place right foot on outside of left knee. Twist to the right, and repeat on other side.

4. *Parivrtta Trikonasana (Rotated Triangle Pose)* (Levels II–III)

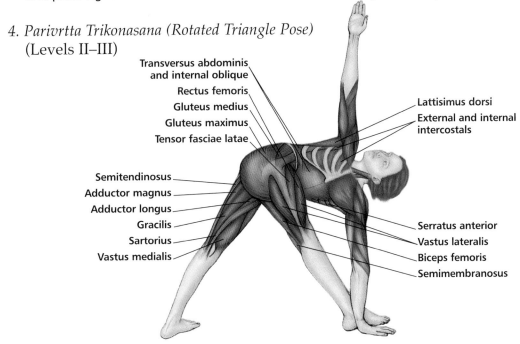

Figure 4.21: Parivrtta trikonasana (rotated triangle pose).

One of the most beneficial Yoga poses, it is much more than a stretch or strength for the obliques. It stimulates the organs, teaches alignment and balance, and extends the limbs. To learn this correctly, take a Yoga class!

5. *The Backbend* (Level III plus)

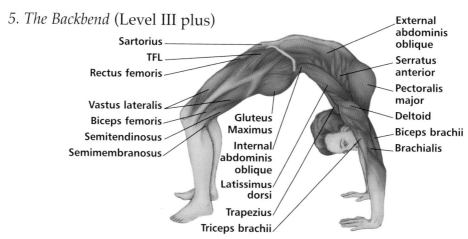

Labels:
Sartorius
TFL
Rectus femoris
Vastus lateralis
Biceps femoris
Semitendinosus
Semimembranosus
Gluteus Maximus
Internal abdominis oblique
Latissimus dorsi
Trapezius
Triceps brachii
External abdominis oblique
Serratus anterior
Pectoralis major
Deltoid
Biceps brachii
Brachialis

Figure 4.22: The backbend (level III plus).

TECHNIQUE

Lie on back, knees bent, feet on floor. With arms bent, place palms flat on floor by the ears. Push hips off floor while trying to extend arms and legs. The spine will hyperextend (arch). Be careful; most people do not need to hyperextend this much.

6. *Swim! Any stroke will stretch the abdominals.*

There are many more stretches for all abdominals. Any body position that rotates, hyperextends or laterally flexes the spine will also stretch the abdominal area. The only spinal position that does not stretch the abdominals is flexion (fetal position).

Many students ask how to exercise the abdominals. Just **use them** and they will strengthen. While driving or sitting at the computer, sit up straight and *tighten* them; while brushing teeth, hold them against the spine; while laying down on the stomach (prone position), pull them up off the floor (do this while watching TV). Be more conscious about what they are doing while standing and talking to someone, or while waiting in line anywhere.

Engage them! The simple act of pulling the abdominals in toward the spine, then up into the ribs and down to the pelvis (without constricting the center too much) lengthens and strengthens them. Do this while walking, running, dancing, cycling, sitting, standing; it will aid in posture and the harmony of the whole body as well.

Remember, working slower may bring more focus to correct muscles and alignment as well as build better strength and endurance than 'racing' through them would. Endless repetition is not necessary, and it is boring. **The best exercise recipe is to:**

1. **Strengthen the muscle, overload it (safely).**
2. **Stretch a muscle, relax to elongate.**
3. **Breathe, and have fun.**

Psoas Major

The **psoas** (do not pronounce the 'p') is the only muscle that connects the upper extremity to the lower extremity, making it a most important postural muscle.

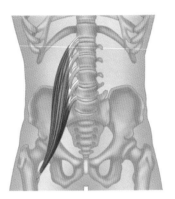

Figure 4.23: Psoas major.

The psoas has a major and a minor muscle, both **synergistic** (they can do the same joint actions at the lumbar spine). The difference is in their attachments: the **major** is the one that connects the femur to the spine (upper to lower extremities); the **minor** connects the pelvis to the spine. Some say the minor will become extinct, as it was important when humans evolved from all four legs to two, and not necessarily needed now. In fact, some people only have it on one side.

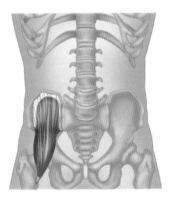

Figure 4.24: Iliacus.

Both psoas'es are part of a larger muscle group called the **iliopsoas**, which also includes the large **iliacus**. This group, contracting simultaneously, flexes the hip. It is the deepest of the hip flexors, making it hard to palpate. The iliacus attaches from the femur to the iliac bone of the pelvis, while the psoas major distally attaches to the femur, and proximally (nearest center) attaches past the hip to the transverse processes of lumbar 1 through 5. The psoas can flex the lumbar spine as well as the hip. If the femur is *fixed* (as in sitting), the iliacus will act on the pelvis, while the psoas will act on the lumbar spine.

The Anatomy of Exercise & Movement

The iliacus can also aid the pelvis in tilting forward; this forward tilt has a tendency to enhance lumbar lordosis (anterior curving) so the psoas, along with another lumbar muscle called the **quadratus lumborum** (see page 68), must be strong enough to stabilize the entire area from too much advanced lordosis, or 'sway back', one of the most common conditions of poor posture. As stated in the beginning of this chapter, the abdominals can also help counteract this.

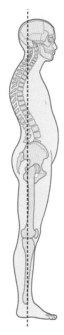

Figure 4.25: Lordotic posture.
Note the exaggerated lumbar curve.

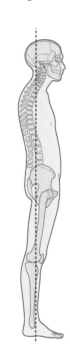

Figure 4.26: Backward tilt of pelvis.

Research suggests that the psoas muscles, by forming a muscle bundle around the lumbar spine with the lower transversospinalis muscles, can also help erect the spine. Either way, as a core muscle the psoas is a major force in correct body alignment. It is also considered an important element in the transfer of weight through the trunk to the legs and feet.

The best way to work the iliopsoas during exercise is to hold the thighs anterior (in front of) the pelvis against gravity. Some sources indicate the iliopsoas can also outwardly rotate the iliofemoral (hip) joint. Adding outward rotation of the thigh to the following exercises will possibly isolate the muscle even more. In these positions, the hip flexors will dominate; the abdominals will stabilize.

Iliopsoas Strengthening Exercises

1. V-Seat (Levels I–III)

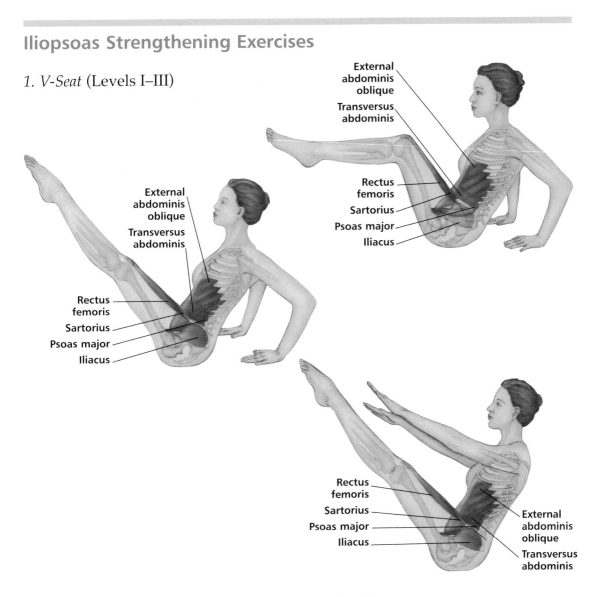

Figure 4.27: V-seat (levels I–III).

TECHNIQUE

Level I: sit just behind 'sit bones', put hands on floor, lean back slightly and raise knees toward chest. Hold for 10 seconds.

Level II: assume position of Level I and try to straighten legs.

Level III: assume position of Level II, and hold arms in front or out to sides (a common gymnastic position, and similar to the **Navasana** (boat pose) in Yoga, and the **Teaser** in Pilates).

2. *The L-Position* (Levels I–III)

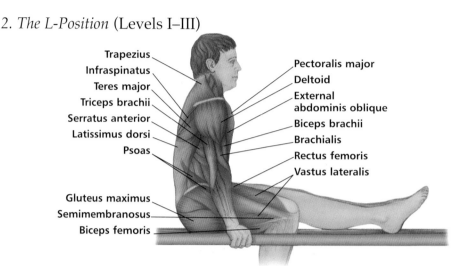

Trapezius
Infraspinatus
Teres major
Triceps brachii
Serratus anterior
Latissimus dorsi
Psoas
Gluteus maximus
Semimembranosus
Biceps femoris

Pectoralis major
Deltoid
External abdominis oblique
Biceps brachii
Brachialis
Rectus femoris
Vastus lateralis

Figure 4.28: L-position (levels I–III).

TECHNIQUE

Level I: with arms supported on a dip machine or parallel bars, lift legs in front with knees bent, and hold for 10 seconds.
Levels II–III: assume position of Level I and straighten legs, holding for 10–30 seconds.

Iliopsoas Stretching Exercises

The iliopsoas is one of the most important muscles to stretch for three reasons:

1) Many humans are becoming a society of hip flexion (sitting). This shortens the hip flexors, which includes the iliopsoas, so stretching will counteract this.

2) If the iliopsoas is short or *tight*, it will cause too much flexion of the hips and the pelvis will tilt forward, causing the lower back muscles to shorten. Over time these muscles will tighten, and atrophy of the abdominals can happen (abdominals tend to relax with forward pelvic tilt). The resulting pronounced lordosis (see page 64), or *sway back*, can lead to lower back problems.

3) Releasing the psoas can stimulate organs, circulation, and movement, affect the nervous and reproductive systems, and relieve sciatic pain and the fear reflex.

To stretch the psoas muscle group, the legs must be extended behind the pelvis. To release it, try the constructive rest position. The **constructive rest position**, sometimes called the horizontal rest position, is a valuable alignment method that enables the skeleton to support the body while muscle tension is released. Lying supine, the knees are bent and resting against each other with the feet wide and turned in. This allows the heavy femurs (thigh bones) to support each other's weight and track nicely into the hip sockets. The spine and pelvis rest neutrally against the floor, while the arms are crossed at the elbows against the chest. The hands hang freely to the sides. Imagery is used to aid the energy flow of the body, relax the breath, and rejuvenate the body.

1. Leg Extensions to the Back (Levels I–III)

TECHNIQUE

Standing, stretch one leg back at a time, knee straight or bent. The 'arabesque' from ballet puts the leg in this position (III). Rotate the leg inward to enhance the stretch.

2. The Psoas Lift (Level I)

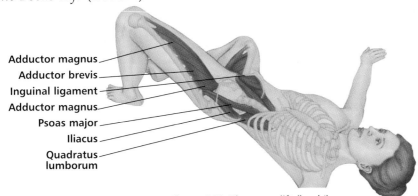

Adductor magnus
Adductor brevis
Inguinal ligament
Adductor magnus
Psoas major
Iliacus
Quadratus lumborum

Figure 4.29: The psoas lift (level I).

TECHNIQUE

Lie on floor with knees bent, feet on floor shoulder-width apart, and arms out for support. Move right leg to one side while feet remain on floor. Lift left hip off the floor and hold the stretch. Repeat on the other side.

3. Advanced Psoas Stretch (Level III plus)
Dhanurasana (Bow Pose)
Similar to full Swan in Pilates

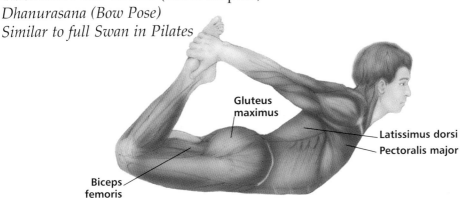

Gluteus maximus

Latissimus dorsi
Pectoralis major

Biceps femoris

Figure 4.30: Pilates swan.

TECHNIQUE

In prone position, bend knees and hold ankles. This will stretch the anterior body quite a bit; care must be taken not to overdo the stretch. This position is advanced because both the spine and shoulders are hyperextending. Support the lower back with the abdominals for added safety.

Feel what is stretching or strengthening, and that the body is responding in a positive manner with no discomfort. Looking inward and sensing kinesthetically what is happening leads to a wiser, deeper, and more balanced workout.

The Anatomy of Exercise & Movement

Quadratus Lumborum

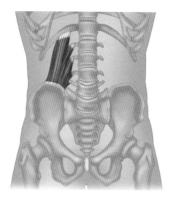

The **quadratus lumborum** is a posterior muscle that covers the lumbar area, from the iliac crest of the pelvis to the transverse processes of the lumbar spine and the 12th rib. It is sometimes referred to as a lateral belly muscle along with the obliques, but not usually considered an abdominal muscle.

Figure 4.31: Quadratus lumborum.

It is mainly a stabilizer of both the lower spine and pelvis, although it can be active in extension and lateral flexion of the spine, and pelvic rotation. As an important stabilizer, it needs to be strong enough to support the alignment of the spine to the pelvis. It can be developed in both stretch and strength exercises that include lateral bending of the spine, or pelvic tilt. It can be stretched during spinal flexion.

Quadratus Lumborum Stretching Exercise

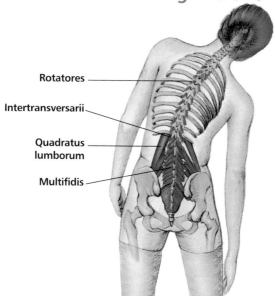

Rotatores

Intertransversarii

Quadratus lumborum

Multifidis

Figure 4.32: Standing lateral side stretch.

TECHNIQUE

Stand with feet about shoulder-width apart and look forward. Keep body upright and slowly bend to the left or right. Reach down leg with hand and do not bend forward.

The Pelvis

The pelvis is a large, circular, bony mass that lies between the spine (upper extremity) and the legs (lower extremity). It is called the 'basin' of the body and since puberty has fused into three bones: two iliac bones and one sacrum.

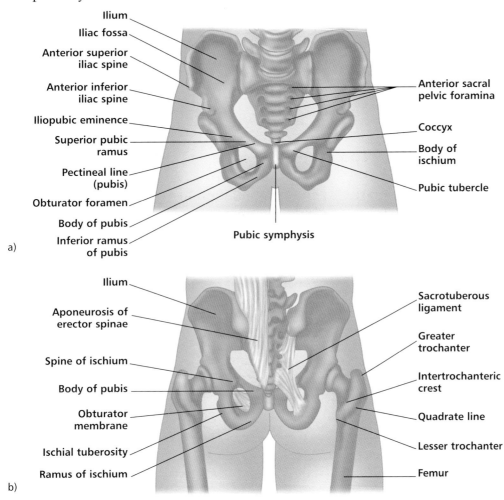

a)

Ilium
Iliac fossa
Anterior superior iliac spine
Anterior inferior iliac spine
Iliopubic eminence
Superior pubic ramus
Pectineal line (pubis)
Obturator foramen
Body of pubis
Inferior ramus of pubis
Pubic symphysis
Anterior sacral pelvic foramina
Coccyx
Body of ischium
Pubic tubercle

b)

Ilium
Aponeurosis of erector spinae
Spine of ischium
Body of pubis
Obturator membrane
Ischial tuberosity
Ramus of ischium
Sacrotuberous ligament
Greater trochanter
Intertrochanteric crest
Quadrate line
Lesser trochanter
Femur

Figure 4.33: Location of the pelvis; a) anterior view, b) posterior view.

The pelvis is a sensitive structure before puberty. Bones are fusing together throughout childhood. Imagine what can happen, therefore, when a younger athlete falls repeatedly on the pelvis, where soft tissue and sutures are still forming into harder surfaces. The only suggestion to this dilemma is to either pad the area heavily, or stop insisting that children become star athletes at such an early age.

The pelvis has two important joint areas, the **sacro-iliac and the iliofemoral joints**. The sacro-iliac is the least moveable joint, where the sacrum and iliac bones articulate. It is considered a gliding joint, very active during child-bearing.

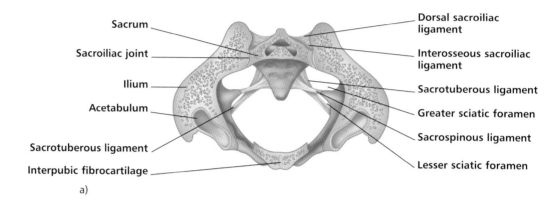

Sacrum

Sacroiliac joint

Ilium

Acetabulum

Sacrotuberous ligament

Interpubic fibrocartilage

Dorsal sacroiliac ligament

Interosseous sacroiliac ligament

Sacrotuberous ligament

Greater sciatic foramen

Sacrospinous ligament

Lesser sciatic foramen

a)

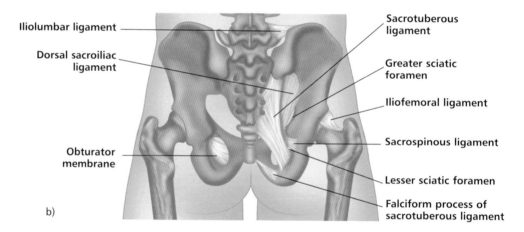

Iliolumbar ligament

Dorsal sacroiliac ligament

Obturator membrane

Sacrotuberous ligament

Greater sciatic foramen

Iliofemoral ligament

Sacrospinous ligament

Lesser sciatic foramen

Falciform process of sacrotuberous ligament

b)

Figure 4.34: The sacro-iliac joint; a) transverse section of the pelvis, b) pelvic ligaments.

There are strong ligaments that connect the two bones. **Ligaments** are somewhat inelastic; once ligaments are overstretched, they are unlikely to bounce back to their original shape. Therefore, it seems reasonable to assume that many women, after childbirth, can experience a sacro-iliac shift because of loosened ligaments. This can cause discomfort in the lower back area that can be addressed through some strength exercises to compensate for the laxity. These exercises also complement the stretch of the six deep rotators of the hip, including the **piriformis**, a muscle that can compress the sciatic nerve and cause pain. These muscles are covered in Chapter 8.

Pelvis Stretching and Strengthening Exercises

1. *Sacro-iliac Joint Stretch* (Level I)

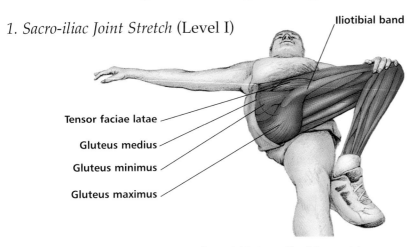

Figure 4.35: Sacro-iliac joint stretch.

TECHNIQUE

Lie on back with bent knees, feet on floor, arms out to side. Cross one ankle over the other knee and roll legs slowly to one side, then the other. Switch legs and repeat.

2. *Sacro-iliac Joint Strength* (Level I)

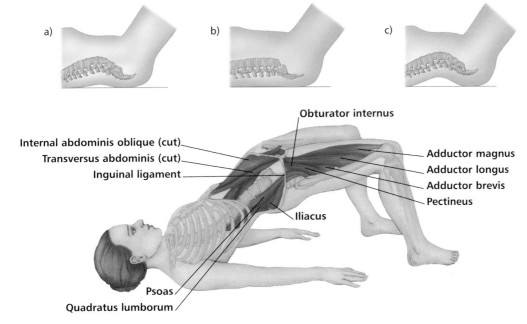

Figure 4.36: Sacro-iliac joint strength (level I). Pelvic tilt (above); a) neutral, where the triangle is parallel to the floor, b) posterior tilt, also known as 'imprint', c) anterior tilt.

TECHNIQUE

This can be done with the tailbone either on or off the floor. Lie on the back with knees bent, and feet on the floor. Allow the pelvis to tilt forward (front hip bones, the ASIS, toward ceiling) then backward (front hip bones toward floor). Concentrate on working deeper abdominals, lower back, and pelvic muscles.

The second joint in the pelvic area, the **iliofemoral**, is the main hip joint. This is the articulation point between the iliac bone and the femur (thigh bone). It is the largest ball-and-socket joint of the body; the femur sits deep in the acetabulum, the socket of the pelvis. Three very large ligaments hold these two bones together, as well as tendons of powerful muscles such as the rectus femoris, a hip flexor and knee extensor. Chapter 8 focuses on this joint specifically.

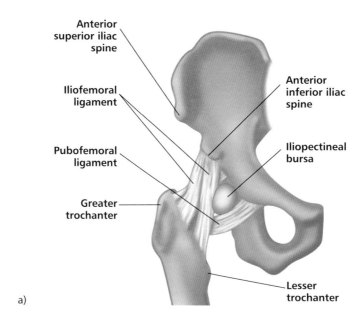

a)

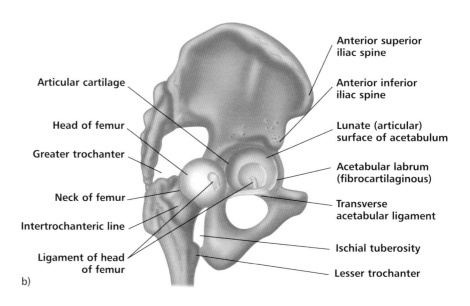

b)

Figure 4.37: The hip joint; a) right leg, anterior view, b) right leg, lateral view.

Besides these two important joint areas where movement can occur, the pelvis *seems* to be able to move on its own. A 'wiggle', or sway of the hips, is actually a rotational movement of the pelvic girdle. This can only happen with help from the lumbar spine, and right and left hip joints. The pelvis can move in all three planes.

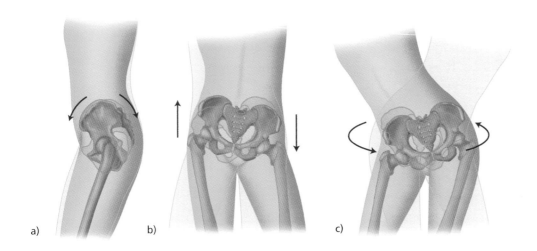

Figure 4.38: The pelvis can move in three planes; a) sagittal, b) frontal, c) horizontal.

Plane 1:
In the sagittal plane, it can move forward and backward, which is usually called pelvic tilt, see page 71. Use the anterior superior iliac spine (ASIS) as a reference point. This point can be felt by placing the hands on the front hip bones. Move the pelvis forward and backward. The lumbar spine will hyperextend and the hips will flex with forward movement of the pelvis. With posterior or backward tilt, the lumbar spine will flex, engaging the psoas and abdominals.

Plane 2:
In the frontal plane, the pelvis will flex laterally and medially, as in 'hiking the hip up'. Some texts refer to lateral flexion right and left; same thing. The lumbar spine will also flex laterally and the hips will abduct and adduct.

Plane 3:
In the horizontal plane, the pelvis rotates inward and outward, although it is very limited and cannot happen without help from the sacro-iliac, lumbar, and hip joints. It is similar to 'twisting'.

One of the most frustrating things in the fields of anatomy and kinesiology is terminology. Various texts refer to the same movements or even muscles with different terms. The above six movements of the pelvis have all been referred to as rotation – if it helps visualize the movement, then why not? What matters is the understanding of the movement.

The Perineal Center

Eric Franklin uses this term in his book, *Pelvic Power*. This is an area of deeper muscles on the pelvic floor, where the central tendon of the diaphragm lies with other muscles such as the sphincter, bulbospongiosus, and perinea. These muscles have important functions during breathing, sex, and childbirth, and are a center for sensitive nerve endings. When stimulated and strengthened, the area can influence energy, sensations, and emotions. Organs like the bladder and kidneys are also affected. One of the best ways to develop this deep center correctly is by lying down with small exercise balls or a soft towel or pillow under the pelvis. This allows the organs to shift upward, releasing their pressure away from the pelvic floor. The person can then lift one or both legs, as in **happy baby** from Yoga, to center and strengthen the area. In **happy baby**, supine position, the knees are bent and separated with thighs against the chest; hands can hold the feet, which are parallel to the ceiling.

Exercises for the pelvic girdle: all levels

1. **Isolations** of the pelvis in jazz dance classes.
2. **Pelvic tilts**, or 'rocks' (see page 71).
3. **Figure 8**: lie on back with knees bent, feet on floor. Raise hips so they are free of the floor, and draw a 'figure 8' with the hips.
4. **Ethnic dance**, such as belly dancing, Hawaiian or Polynesian dancing, and/or African dance.

Have fun whilst exercising! I have not met anyone who did not have fun in a jazz or ethnic movement class.

Beware of lower back positions – support the lumbar spine with the abdominals, psoas, and quadratus lumborum.

Myths of the Core Dispelled

It is not only the abdominals

The central core is stabilized by all FOUR abdominals, as well as the psoas major, quadratus lumborum, erector spinae muscle group, even the latissimus dorsi, rhomboids, and the trapezius muscles because of their proximity to the spine. These muscles 'girdle' the spine, giving it support and the freedom to move. Deeper, smaller muscle bundles also have a profound effect on posture, such as the transversospinalis and intertransverse posterior muscles of the spine, allowing it to lengthen, bend, twist, and curve naturally. **The suppleness and conditioning of all the core muscles in balance with each other is most important in providing stability for the spine as it supports body movement.**

"Naval to spine" is only an image

This visualization can help many people to engage the deepest abdominal, the transversus abdominis, which is a great stabilizer of the lower torso. However, it must be stated that while 'bringing the naval toward the spine', one must envision length of the abdominals against the spine, from the lower sternum to the pubic bone. This method negates the 'crunch' and lengthens the abdominals to support the spine, therefore relieving stress and compression of the lumbar area. **All core muscles need to be addressed in workouts, not concentration on just one; this would lead to imbalance.**

The six-pack is not that important

The rectus abdominis and its three tendinous intersections (on each side make six!) are visible when the muscle contracts. This muscle, in constant contraction, would lead to imbalance. **It is not the look, but strength and correct use that counts.**

Main Muscles Involved in Movements of the Thoracic/Lumbar Spine

Flexion
Muscles of Anterior Abdominal Wall; Psoas Major and Minor

Extension
Erector Spinae; Quadratus Lumborum; Longus Colli; Interspinalis; Intertransversarii; Multifidis; Rotatores; Semispinalis Thoracis

Rotation and Lateral Flexion
Iliocostalis Lumborum; Iliocostalis Thoracis; Multifidis; Rotatores; Intertransversarii; Quadratus Lumborum; Muscles of Anterior Abdominal Wall

Chapter

5

The Shoulder Region

The shoulder region is actually composed of five joints: the sternoclavicular (SC) joint, the acromioclavicular (AC) joint, the coracoclavicular joint, the glenohumeral joint, and the scapulothoracic joint, where the shoulder-blade glides on the chest wall. The articulation referred to specifically as the shoulder joint is the glenohumeral joint, whereas the other articulations are joints of the shoulder girdle.

The structure of the shoulder permits a wide range of motion, allowing the positioning of the arm and hand. Movements of the shoulder region are determined by muscles that are located on the chest, back, and upper arms. Therefore, whatever the shoulder region is doing determines the look of the majority of the upper extremity.

The movements of the arms are what will shape most of the back muscles, as well as the chest and arm. Other muscles in these areas are contoured by movements of the scapula, the shoulder girdle joint area.

Glenohumeral Joint

This is the main shoulder joint, specifically the articulation between the scapula and the humerus. A multi-axial ball-and-socket joint, the head of the humerus (ball) sits in the glenoid cavity (socket). The socket is shallow compared to other ball-and-socket joints; this allows for greater range of motion, but the joint is less stable because of it. The head of the humerus is larger than the cavity it fits into. To help it fit tighter there is a fibro-cartilaginous ring called the **glenoid labrum** that helps seal the humerus in place more snugly.

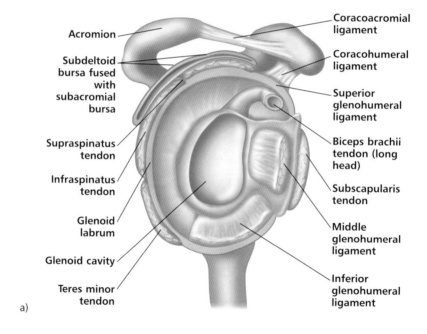

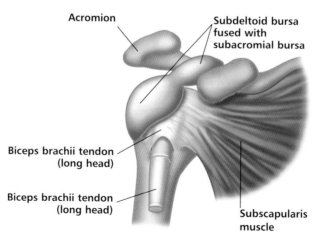

Figure 5.1: The glenohumeral joint; a) right arm, lateral view, b) right arm, anterior view (cut).

Shoulder Joint Ligaments

Because the shoulder joint articulation is not deep and gravity acts as a force on the humerus, the ligaments of the joint must be very strong and intact to help hold the joint together. There are three glenohumeral ligaments in the front of the joint, and an inferior and superior coracohumeral ligament (running from the coracoid to the humerus) that are the main reinforcing structures.

The shoulder joint capsule is strengthened with the semicircular humeri, a ligamentous tissue that lies in close relationship with the tendons of the rotator cuff to bring integrity to the area.

Movements of the Shoulder Joint

Different texts indicate more actions at the shoulder joint than others. The main actions are the true ball-and-socket joint actions of **flexion, extension, abduction, adduction, internal (medial)** and **external (lateral) rotation**. Because the joint is so mobile (thanks to the aid of the shoulder girdle joint area) the joint can also hyper-flex, hyper-extend, hyper-abduct and hyper-adduct. Add another true joint action of moving the humerus from the frontal plane to the sagittal plane and back again, and **horizontal adduction/abduction** is included. Diagonal movements are some of these actions combined.

Note: the shoulder joint action of horizontal adduction is also sometimes called horizontal flexion; the action of horizontal abduction can also be referred to as horizontal extension.

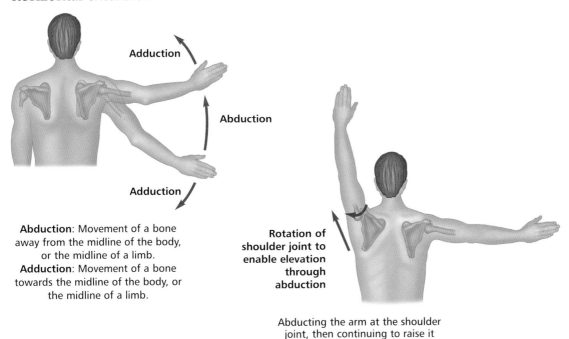

Abduction: Movement of a bone away from the midline of the body, or the midline of a limb.
Adduction: Movement of a bone towards the midline of the body, or the midline of a limb.

Abducting the arm at the shoulder joint, then continuing to raise it above the head in the frontal plane can be referred to as **elevation through abduction**.

The Anatomy of Exercise & Movement

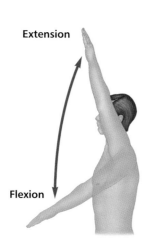

Extension

Flexion

Extension: To straighten or bend backward away from the foetal position.
Flexion: Bending to decrease the angle between bones at a joint. From the anatomical position, flexion is usually forward, except at the knee joint where it is backward. The way to remember this is that flexion is always toward the foetal position.

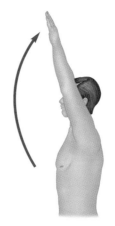

Flexing the arm at the shoulder joint, then continuing to raise it above the head in the sagittal plane can be referred to as **elevation through flexion**.

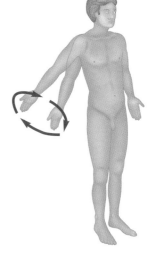

Circumduction: Movement in which the distal end of a bone moves in a circle, while the proximal end remains stable; the movement combines flexion, abduction, extension, and adduction.

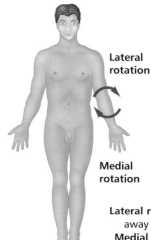

Lateral rotation

Medial rotation

Lateral rotation: To turn out, away from the midline.
Medial rotation: To turn in towards the midline.

Figure 5.2: Movements of the shoulder joint.

Shoulder Joint Muscles

Muscles that move the upper arm have to cross the glenohumeral joint to work it; this is a major principle of kinesiology: if a muscle does not cross from one of the articulated bones to the other, how can the joint be moved?

Example: the infraspinatus muscle crosses the shoulder joint from the scapula to the humerus to work it.

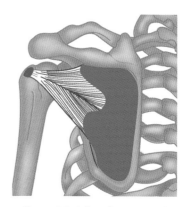

Figure 5.3: Infraspinatus muscle.

Anteriorly the muscles that cross the shoulder joint are the **pectoralis major, anterior deltoid, coracobrachialis,** and **biceps brachii.** Posterior muscles are the **supraspinatus, infraspinatus, teres major and minor, latissimus dorsi, posterior deltoid,** and **triceps brachii.** The **subscapularis** rounds out the shoulder joint's eleven muscles, hidden behind the rib cage and on the anterior side of the scapula. The tendons of these muscles cross the shoulder joint from one bone to the other.

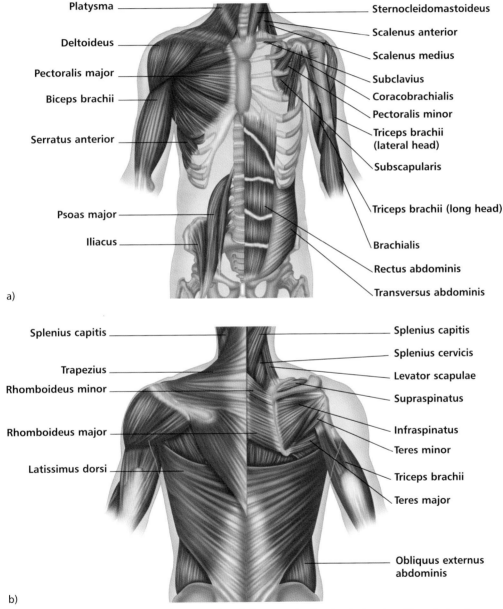

Figure 5.4: Superficial and intermediate muscles of the upper body; a) anterior view, b) posterior view.

The shoulder joint is complicated, multi-faceted and 'multi-muscled'. This section will focus on the three largest muscles of the joint, as well as the rotator cuff muscles.

Deltoids

Multipennate is defined as a muscle that has several tendons with fibers running diagonally between them, similar to a feather. The deltoid is an example. Superficially capping the shoulder, the deltoid is divided into three parts: anterior, middle, and posterior.

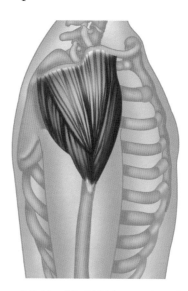

Figure 5.5: The deltoid (right arm, lateral view).

The proximal front fibers begin on the clavicle, the middle on the acromion process of the scapula, and the back on the spine of the scapula, all coming together as the deltoid muscle belly gives the shoulder its round shape. The distal attachment is joined together on the humerus at the deltoid tuberosity.

When all three sections contract simultaneously they abduct the arm, bringing it out from the side and up in the frontal plane. Most lifting movements involve the deltoids.

The fun happens when trying to decipher the differences. The anterior deltoid can flex the arm, while the posterior extends it. These are opposite actions in the same plane (sagittal), which seems impossible in the same muscle. However, the location, or path of the fibers, explains it. The front deltoid can also inward rotate while the posterior outward rotates, and can horizontally adduct while the posterior horizontally abducts. The middle deltoid is the least complicated; it only abducts, synergistic with the supraspinatus muscle.

Such a complicated muscle also acts as a shock absorber, protecting the shoulder from impact. It does not act on any joint other than the shoulder. Since it is so visible, it is a popular muscle in the weight room.

Deltoid Strengthening Exercises

Lateral raises, overhead presses. To isolate different parts, take the arm through all actions, using dumbbells.

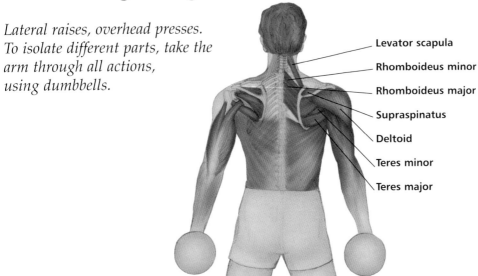

- Levator scapula
- Rhomboideus minor
- Rhomboideus major
- Supraspinatus
- Deltoid
- Teres minor
- Teres major

Figure 5.6: Dumbbell standing lateral raise.

TECHNIQUE

Stand with feet shoulder-width apart. Spine neutral, knees soft, dumbbells in hand at sides. Maintaining a fixed elbow angle of about 10 degrees, raise the arms laterally to shoulder height. Keep the wrist, elbow and shoulder in line. Lower and repeat.

Deltoid Stretching Exercise

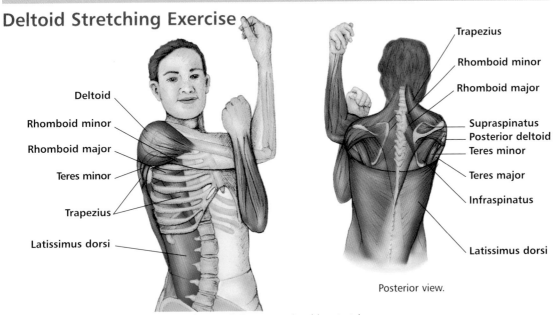

- Deltoid
- Rhomboid minor
- Rhomboid major
- Teres minor
- Trapezius
- Latissimus dorsi

- Trapezius
- Rhomboid minor
- Rhomboid major
- Supraspinatus
- Posterior deltoid
- Teres minor
- Teres major
- Infraspinatus
- Latissimus dorsi

Posterior view.

Figure 5.7: Bent arm shoulder stretch.

TECHNIQUE

Stand upright and place one arm across the body. Bend the arm at 90 degrees and pull the elbow towards the opposite shoulder. Keep the upper arm parallel to the ground. See figure 5.10 for anterior deltoid stretch.

Pectoralis Major

Called the 'chest' muscle, the pectoralis major covers the front of the upper body from the clavicle, sternum, and ribs 1 through 6 to the humerus. Depending on which text is used, this muscle has either two or three sections. Two areas are described as clavicular and sternal, three are upper, middle, and lower.

Another multipennate muscle, the pectoralis major works only the shoulder joint. The pectoralis minor located under the major actually works a different joint, the shoulder girdle, explained in the next section.

The pectoralis major has an interesting 'twist': as it attaches distally to the humerus, the tendons of the two sections rotate, so that the top portion of the tendon (clavicular) ends up below the sternal portion on the humerus.

The twist of the tendon allows the action of inward rotation, as does a twist from the latissimus dorsi posteriorly. The other prominent action from both sections of the pectoralis major is horizontal adduction, or bringing the arms from the side to the front (frontal to sagittal planes).

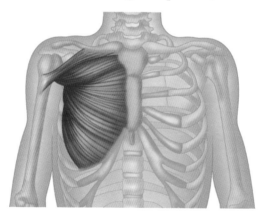

Figure 5.8: The pectoralis major.

The two sections differ in the sagittal plane: the clavicular head flexes, while the sternal portion extends. This is hard to understand from a mechanical point of view, since the entire pectoralis major is noted as an anterior muscle. Usually muscles located anteriorly can only do actions toward the front of the body; extension is an action that is posterior, returning to or behind the body.

To further complicate the muscle, when the upper arm is 90 degrees (out to the side at shoulder level) the clavicular section can raise it higher by abducting. It can also lower it (adduction) along with the sternal portion, below 90 degrees.

Pectoralis Major Strengthening Exercises

Bench press, push-ups, throwing a ball, swimming, tennis.

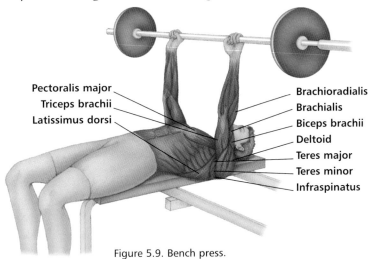

Pectoralis major
Triceps brachii
Latissimus dorsi

Brachioradialis
Brachialis
Biceps brachii
Deltoid
Teres major
Teres minor
Infraspinatus

Figure 5.9. Bench press.

TECHNIQUE

Lie on a bench and hold a barbell above the chest with arms directly above the collar bone. Arms extended, feet flat, and spine neutral. Grip the bar with the hands wider than the shoulders; inhale and lower the barbell towards the chest. Exhale, extending the arms to push up to the ceiling, and return to the starting position.

Pectoralis Major Stretching Exercise

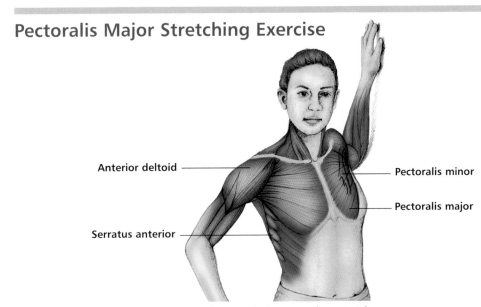

Anterior deltoid

Serratus anterior

Pectoralis minor

Pectoralis major

Figure 5.10: Bent arm chest stretch.

TECHNIQUE

Stand with the arm extended and the forearm at 90 degrees to the ground. Rest the forearm against an immoveable object and turn shoulders and body away from the extended arm.

Latissimus Dorsi

The 'lats', as they are called, cover most of the mid to lower back. The term means 'widest back muscle'. It travels from the thoracic spinal processes of T7–T12 to the sacral and iliac crests, then across to the humerus.

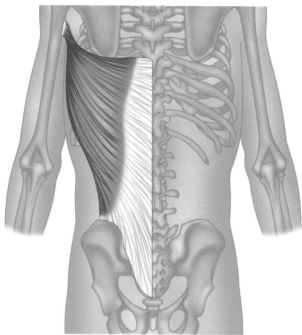

Its main actions are extension, adduction, and inward (medial) rotation of the shoulder joint. It is also a strong assistor, in horizontal abduction while inward rotating, and in raising the thorax toward the arm in pull-ups. This is an extremely powerful muscle, bringing anything in towards the body. It is very active in climbing, rowing, swimming, gymnastics events, even lifting a suitcase

Figure 5.11: Latissimus dorsi..

Latissimus Dorsi Strengthening Exercises

Pull-ups, chin-ups, lat. pull-downs, rowing machines.

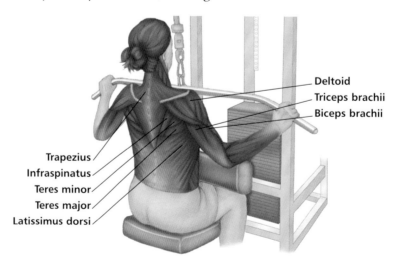

Deltoid
Triceps brachii
Biceps brachii

Trapezius
Infraspinatus
Teres minor
Teres major
Latissimus dorsi

Figure 5.12: Lat. pull-downs.

TECHNIQUE

Sit with the thighs tucked under the pad, and use a wide, palm-out grip to hold the bar. Keeping the trunk still, pull the bar downward until it touches the chest. Return to the starting position.

Latissimus Dorsi Stretching Exercises

Down dog, kneeling reach forward stretch, child's pose.

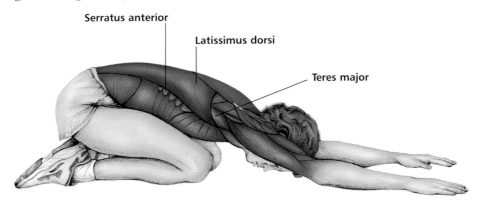

Figure 5.13: Kneeling reach forward stretch.

TECHNIQUE

Kneel on the ground and reach forward with hands. Let the head fall forward and push the buttocks toward feet.

The Rotator Cuff

The name is deceiving: rotation is not the primary function of the rotator cuff muscles.

The rotator cuff's main purpose is to stabilize the head of the humerus within the glenoid cavity; in other words, hold the arm in place.

This is mainly done by the tendons of the four rotator cuff muscles of the glenohumeral joint: **supraspinatus, infraspinatus, teres minor,** and **subscapularis** (commonly referred to as "**SITS**" muscles). These muscles are small in comparison to other shoulder joint muscles, yet must be strong enough to endure repeated movements of the arm, especially forward and/or overhead. How many times does someone throw, reach, or lift something? These movements are a part of everyday life, and specifically important in many sports: swimming, baseball, weight-lifting, golf, etc. Over-stress of these tendons can produce inflammation or tears (partial or full) resulting in pain and injury to the rotator cuff. Prevention is the best key to survival: exercising the cuff before injury will strengthen the joint area.

The subacromial bursa (a fluid-filled sac), provides the rotator cuff with lubrication to assist movement (see figure 5.1a). This is the largest and most commonly injured bursa in the shoulder region, because of continued stress on the rotator cuff muscles. Overuse is the main cause of an inflamed bursa.

The Anatomy of Exercise & Movement

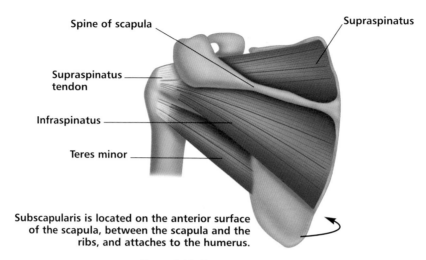

Spine of scapula

Supraspinatus

Supraspinatus tendon

Infraspinatus

Teres minor

Subscapularis is located on the anterior surface of the scapula, between the scapula and the ribs, and attaches to the humerus.

Figure 5.14: The rotator cuff muscles.

Rotator Cuff Strengthening Exercises

The four cuff muscles do actions that, when combined together, are abduction, inward rotation, outward rotation, extension, and horizontal abduction of the shoulder joint. The following are exercises that do these actions, therefore strengthening the muscles:

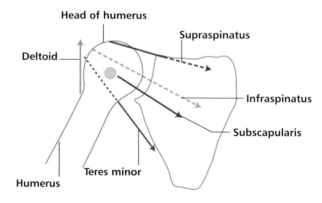

Head of humerus

Supraspinatus

Deltoid

Infraspinatus

Subscapularis

Teres minor

Humerus

Figure 5.15: Directions of rotator cuff muscle action.

1. *Lateral Raises* (Level I) (see figure 5.6)
   Abduction by deltoids and **supraspinatus**

   TECHNIQUE

   Using weights or therabands in hands to add more resistance, begin with arms down at sides and lift them out and up to shoulder level. Hold for 10 counts, then lower slowly. Repeat at least 3 times.

2. *Lateral Raises with Inward/Outward Rotation* (Level I)
This works all four rotator cuff muscles plus the deltoids

TECHNIQUE

While performing lateral raises, rotate arms forward and backward, elbow straight or bent. The forearm goes forward for inward rotation and backward for outward rotation. Doing one arm at a time can be beneficial, as the stronger arm will not take over.

3. *Bent-over Lateral Raises (Reverse Flyes)* (Level II)
Horizontal extension – **infraspinatus and teres minor**

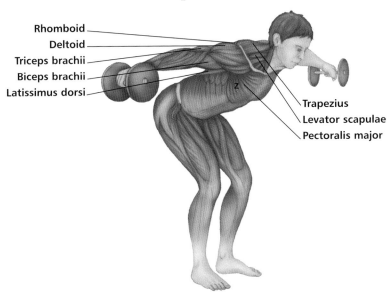

Rhomboid
Deltoid
Triceps brachii
Biceps brachii
Latissimus dorsi

Trapezius
Levator scapulae
Pectoralis major

Figure 5.16: The bent-over lateral raise.

TECHNIQUE

Assume position of the first exercise, lateral raises. Bend forward at the waist with knees slightly bent and abdominals supporting the spine. Take arms toward floor then raise them out to the side. This change in body position allows the action of horizontal extension (sometimes called *horizontal abduction*). This works two of the rotators: the teres minor and infraspinatus. The latissimus dorsi and teres major also do this action, but are not part of the rotator cuff. To isolate the two cuff muscles, slightly outward rotate.

4. *Dumbbell Press* (Level II)
Abduction and rotation, **working all four cuff muscles**

TECHNIQUE

Sit with the back straight, holding dumbbells in hands with arms out at sides and elbows bent. Raise and lower arms for abduction; roll arms forward and back for rotation. To add horizontal extension, take the arms behind the shoulders. **Rotational action towards the back (external, or outward rotation of shoulder) is a must for rotator cuff conditioning, and great for golfers, who need to stretch and strengthen!**

5. *Extensions* (depending on weights) (Level I–III)
"Kickbacks".

TECHNIQUE

Stand with one foot in front of the other for balance, with knees slightly bent. Bend forward at the waist keeping the back straight. While holding on to front knee with the same side hand, take other arm behind and up. Repeat 8–12 times, in sets, to fatigue the muscles.

6. *Swimming (all strokes)*

TECHNIQUE

The **backstroke** and **breaststroke** in swimming work rotation, circumduction (a combination of flexion, extension, abduction and adduction), and horizontal extension respectively. This is a nearly complete workout for the shoulder joint – try to outward rotate while doing the backstroke for variety.

The **butterfly** emphasizes internal rotation to the extreme (against water resistance while propelling the body forward). This can cause damage to the cuff unless correct conditioning is done: **strengthen and stretch the shoulder even in the 'off season'.**

Rotator Cuff Stretching Exercise

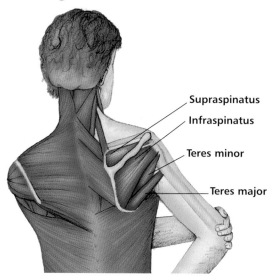

- Supraspinatus
- Infraspinatus
- Teres minor
- Teres major

Figure 5.17: Elbow-out rotator stretch.

TECHNIQUE

Stand with one hand behind the middle of the back and elbow pointing out. Reach over with the other hand and gently pull elbow forward. Refer to figure 5.10 to stretch the anterior rotator cuff muscle, the subscapularis.

Shoulder Girdle Joint

The shoulder girdle is a separate joint area that allows the shoulder joint to achieve its great range of motion. Three bones articulate at two different areas to form the shoulder girdle: the clavicle, scapula, and sternum. Movements of the shoulder girdle are activated mostly at the **sternoclavicular joint**, which in turn moves the scapula. This is the only point where the axial skeleton connects to the trunk.

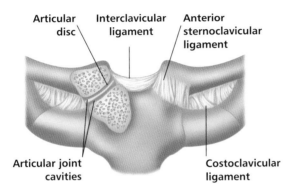

Figure 5.18: The sternoclavicular joint (anterior view). Note that posterior aspect of joint has a posterior sternoclavicular ligament similar, but weaker, than anterior sternoclavicular ligament.

Movements of the Shoulder Girdle

There are eight actions of the shoulder girdle, depending again on what text is referred to (see figure 5.19). For purposes of this book the movements listed are the ones most associated with exercise. They are **elevation, depression, abduction (protraction) and adduction (retraction), upward and downward rotation, and forward and backward tilt.** The actions are indicated by how the scapula moves in space: the scapula moving up is elevation, down is depression; away from the spine, abduction and toward the spine, adduction. Upward rotation is accomplished by the scapula's inferior angle moving out and up, downward rotation is the return from this position. Forward tilt is best seen when the arm is extended behind the body, and backward tilt can happen in a backbend, where the superior scapula tips posteriorly.

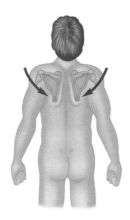

Retraction: Movement backwards in the transverse plane, as in bracing the shoulder girdle back, military style.

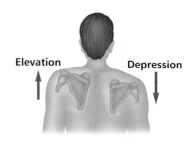

Elevation   Depression

Elevation: Movement of a part of the body upward along the frontal plane. For example, elevating the scapula by shrugging the shoulders.
Depression: Movement of an elevated part of the body downward to its original position.

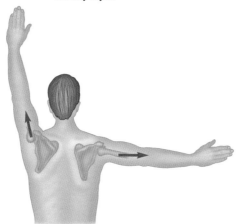

Upward rotation: Scapula's inferior angle moving up and out.
Downward rotation: Return from this position.

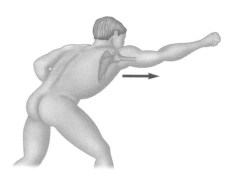

Protraction: Movement forward in the transverse plane. For example, protraction of the shoulder girdle, as in rounding the shoulder.

Figure 5.19: Movements of the shoulder girdle joint.

Shoulder Girdle Muscles

The six muscles working the girdle are the **pectoralis minor, serratus anterior, subclavius, levator scapula, rhomboids,** and **trapezius** (see figure 5.4). All six muscles are located on the chest anteriorly or the back posteriorly. Two of them, the levator scapula and the upper trapezius, are biarticulate with the cervical spine. The largest muscle, the trapezius, is worthy of explanation, as its parts are very specific.

Trapezius

FOUR parts in some texts, three in others. The "traps", as they are called, cover the upper back in a semi-diamond shape, its longest section reaching from the skull down to the last thoracic vertebra. The width is also impressive, going from the outside of one shoulder to the other. Although large, it mainly works one joint: the shoulder girdle. It can aid other joints in breathing or stability, but it essentially lifts, depresses, rotates, or brings the scapula closer to the spine as part of the girdle. The name is derived from the Latin *'trapezium', or 'the shape of the muscle paired'*; a quadrilateral with no parallel sides. It too is so specialized that it can do opposite actions in the same plane.

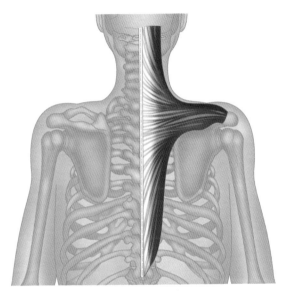

Figure 5.20: Trapezius.

With the trapezius muscle, it is best to list the parts and their specific actions:

Part I (upper): elevation of scapula, extension of head
Part II (mid): elevation, upward rotation, adduction
Part III: adduction
Part IV (lower): depression, upward rotation, adduction

When the trapezius contracts simultaneously, the strong action is adduction, bringing the scapula closer to the spine with help from the rhomboids. These muscles are active in correct posture, and used when lifting heavy objects. The middle and lower trap can also upward rotate, bringing the bottom of the scapula out and up. This is done in combination with raising the arms out to the side. Parts I & II also raise the scapula straight up, lifting the shoulders as in a shoulder shrug, while Part IV presses the shoulders straight down.

Since the trapezius is large and superficial, it is a strong focus in weight lifting and toning. The upper part of the muscle is affected when stressed, as the shoulders become tight because of tension, physically and/or emotionally.

The connection between energy, connective tissue and muscle contraction is just now being scientifically recognized.

Trapezius Strengthening Exercises

Bent-over lateral raises, upright rows, rowing machines, elevation for upper area, with adduction.

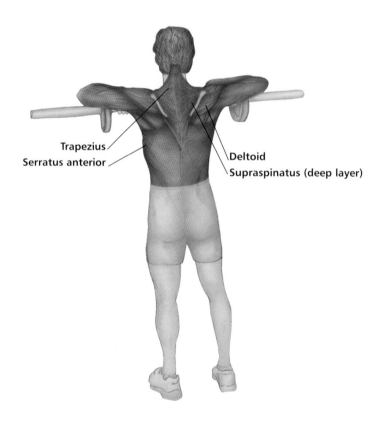

Figure 5.21: Upright rows.

TECHNIQUE

Hold the barbell, using a palm-down grip with hands slightly narrower than shoulder-width apart, arms extended down. Pull hands vertically upward to the upper chest, keeping elbows high. Slowly return to the starting position. **Caution: upright rows can compromise the anterior deltoid if the shoulders are raised too high; depression of the scapula should be emphasized.**

Trapezius Stretching Exercise

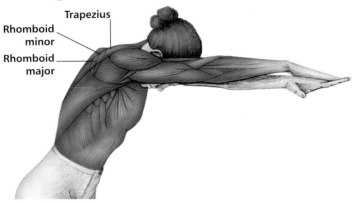

Trapezius

Rhomboid minor

Rhomboid major

Figure 5.22: Reaching upper back stretch.

TECHNIQUE

Stand with the arms out in front and crossed over. Push the hands forward as far as possible and let the head fall forward. Concentrate on reaching forward with the hands, and separating the shoulder-blades. *For the upper part of trapezius, stretch head from side to side.*

Summary: The Shoulder Joint and Girdle Combined

The seventeen muscles united from these two joint areas contract to work the most flexible, yet unstable, part of the body. Flexible because it can do many actions (think how the arm can move in so many directions); this is because the joint and girdle work together to allow for a greater range of motion. When the humerus rises to the side (abduction of the shoulder joint) the arm would only be able to lift to shoulder level because the humerus hits the acromion process of the scapula. The shoulder girdle joint then upward rotates to lift the scapula so the humerus can go higher. The same happens in shoulder joint flexion: the arm (humerus) rises in the sagittal plane, and hits the acromion process; scapula actions allow the arm to rise higher.

The area is unstable, as stated before, because the glenoid cavity is not deep enough for the humerus to fit inside it. Gravity and other forces make the tendons and ligaments work hard to hold the head of the humerus in place, or *stabilize the joint*. The shoulder region is truly unique.

More Shoulder Strengthening Exercises

There are many other exercises that can work the shoulder muscles. The **push-up**, against resistance (gravity), strengthens the pectoralis major, pectoralis minor, serratus anterior, anterior deltoid, coracobrachialis, biceps brachii, and triceps brachii. Add the abdominals by engaging them to support the spine, whether knees are bent or straight. Keep the elbows close to the body.

Dips are one of the best exercises for the arms and shoulder, and can be done with or without bars or bench. They strengthen the front muscles of the shoulder joint (pectoralis major, anterior deltoid) and the back muscles of the elbow joint, the triceps brachii and anconeus. They also concentrically contract the abductors and posterior tilters of the shoulder girdle, the pectoralis minor and the serratus anterior. The triceps brachii are especially challenged.

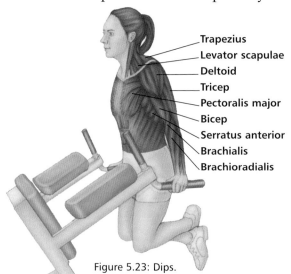

Trapezius
Levator scapulae
Deltoid
Tricep
Pectoralis major
Bicep
Serratus anterior
Brachialis
Brachioradialis

Figure 5.23: Dips.

Hold the bars with arms extended and chest leaning forward. Bend elbows to 90 degrees and lower body. Return to start position. If no bars or machines are available, put body in supine position on the floor with arms extended under shoulders, and hips off the floor. Bend and straighten elbows. In levels I–II, the knees are bent with feet on the floor. Level III is legs straight.

In Yoga, the **upward** and **downward facing dog** (see Chapter 3, figures 3.14/3.15) are great shoulder strength and stabilizer positions. The **down dog** hyper-flexes the shoulder joint and adducts and depresses the shoulder girdle. This involves the anterior shoulder joint muscles, and the posterior trapezius and rhomboids of the girdle, as well as the subclavius. The **up dog** also adducts the shoulder girdle, and works the shoulder joint in stabilization, isometrically contracting the extensors.

The Yoga **plank** position is an isometric push-up, and similar to the **front support** in Pilates. Both exercises can be lowered slowly to the floor to eccentrically contract the flexors of the shoulder joint, abductors of the shoulder girdle, and extensors of the elbow. These same muscles concentrically contract on the way up from the floor, against gravity. A Yoga **reverse plank** (similar to **horizontal dip** but with straight arms) is a great exercise for stabilizing the shoulder area. Care must be taken as the arm is in a hyperextended position, and the scapula is forward tilting.

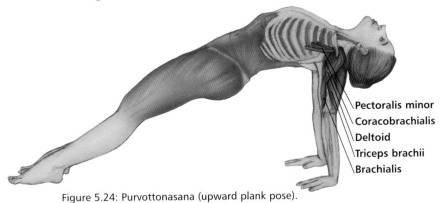

Pectoralis minor
Coracobrachialis
Deltoid
Triceps brachii
Brachialis

Figure 5.24: Purvottonasana (upward plank pose).

TECHNIQUE

Sit and place hands on floor several inches behind hips, fingers pointing forward. With either bent or straight knees, press the feet and hands down into the floor and lift the hips. Keep shoulder-blades against and down the back to lift the chest. Leave head in line with spine to keep the neck from hyperextending too much. This exercise is ideal as a 'heart opener', stretching the anterior side of the body.

More Shoulder Stretching Exercises

There is usually not enough attention given to stretching the muscles around the shoulder. Many people focus on strength, whether for the look, or to perform better, disregarding a stretch routine. Without stretch, muscles may bulk; this can limit flexibility. Remember that stretching elongates the muscles, allowing for better range of motion of joints, which is the definition of flexibility.

Having a freer range of motion with adequate strength training can prevent injury.

Stretching is simple and quick, and most effective when done after a hard workout. Exercises listed are all easy and can be done by anyone. Those people who have worked the upper extremity to enormous proportions will have trouble because their muscles will 'get in the way'. I have had students who are not able to do the first exercise because they cannot touch a hand to the same shoulder – the tricep is tight and the bicep too large!

Bent Arm Circles

TECHNIQUE

Place right hand on right shoulder, left hand on left shoulder, and circle the elbows to the fullest range of motion, ten circles in each direction.

Side Stretches

TECHNIQUE

Clasp hands in front of chest and turn them 'inside out'. Lift arms above head, keeping shoulders down, then stretch to the right and left. Keep elbows straight, if possible.

Towel Stretches

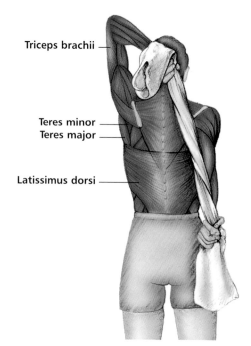

Triceps brachii

Teres minor
Teres major

Latissimus dorsi

Figure 5.25: Towel stretch.

TECHNIQUE

Take a towel, strap, or band, put an end in each hand, and move arms in front and behind to the fullest range of motion.

Myths of the Shoulder Dispelled

Working the 'lats' does not mean the back

Countless students have related how they are exercising the back to work their lats. The back is not a joint; the latissimus dorsi is located posteriorly on the back of the upper extremity, but works the shoulder joint. If it needs to be strengthened, it must adduct, extend, inward rotate, or horizontally abduct the humerus (upper arm) as part of the shoulder joint. The 'lats' do not work the spine or shoulder girdle, which are the only joint areas in the back - they work the shoulder. **The latissimus dorsi works the shoulder joint, not the spine.**

Shoulder dislocation and separation are not the same

Dislocation is where the humerus and the scapula are actually out of articulation with each other. Separation is usually when the acromion process of the scapula and the clavicle come apart at the acromio-clavicular joint. **The true shoulder joint is the articulation between the humerus and the glenoid cavity of the scapula, which moves the arm.**

A frozen shoulder can be unfrozen

Many people suffer from a condition known as 'frozen shoulder', which can range from inflammation and pain, to complete immobility. The ligaments become inflamed and limit range of motion, or there may be scar tissue build up that negates movement. **Treatment can range anywhere from anti-inflammatory methods, to physical therapy and/or possible surgery, but it is treatable.**

People do not have the same range of motion in the shoulder

Range of motion can be limited by the following factors: bone structure, ligament elasticity, muscle condition, injury, even nutrition. **Range of motion at any joint is highly individual.**

The Anatomy of Exercise & Movement

Main Muscles Involved in Movements of the Shoulder Region

Shoulder Joint

Flexion
Deltoideus (anterior portion); Pectoralis Major (clavicular portion : sternocostal portion flexes the extended humerus as far as the position of rest); Biceps Brachii; Coracobrachialis

Extension
Deltoideus (posterior portion); Teres Major (of flexed humerus); Latissimus Dorsi (of flexed humerus); Pectoralis Major (sternocostal portion of flexed humerus); Triceps Brachii (long head to position of rest); Teres Minor; Infraspinatus

Abduction
Deltoideus; Supraspinatus; Biceps Brachii (long head; weak action); Pectoralis Major (clavicular head) above 90 degrees

Adduction
Pectoralis Major; Teres Major; Latissimus Dorsi; Triceps Brachii (long head); Coracobrachialis (weak)

Lateral Rotation
Deltoideus (posterior portion); Infraspinatus; Teres Minor

Medial Rotation
Pectoralis Major; Teres Major; Latissimus Dorsi; Deltoideus (anterior portion); Subscapularis

Horizontal Flexion (Horizontal Adduction)
Deltoideus (anterior portion); Pectoralis Major; Subscapularis, Biceps Brachii; Coracobrachialis

Horizontal Extension (Horizontal Abduction)
Deltoideus (posterior portion); Infraspinatus; Teres Minor; Latissimus Dorsi and Teres Major when shoulder is outward rotated

Shoulder Girdle

Elevation
Trapezius (upper fibers); Levator Scapulae; Rhomboideus Minor; Rhomboideus Major

Depression
Trapezius (lower fibers); Pectoralis Minor; Subclavius

Protraction (Abduction)
Serratus Anterior; Pectoralis Minor

Anterior Tilt
Pectoralis Minor

Retraction (Adduction)
Trapezius (middle and lower fibers); Rhomboideus Minor; Rhomboideus Major

Lateral Displacement of Inferior Angle of Scapula (Upward Rotation)
Serratus Anterior; Trapezius (middle and lower fibers)

Medial Displacement of Inferior Angle of Scapula (Downward Rotation)
Pectoralis Minor; Rhomboideus Minor; Rhomboideus Major

6

The Elbow and Radio-Ulnar Joints

The Elbow Joint

The elbow joint is comprised of the humerus (upper arm bone) and radius and ulna (the two forearm bones, with the ulna being the most medial). At the distal end of the humerus are the trochlea and the capitulum, which together form part of the elbow joint with the radius and ulna.

The Radio-ulnar Joint

Often confused with the elbow joint, the radio-ulnar joint is a separate rotary joint, classified as a pivot joint. It is uni-axial, working in the horizontal/transverse plane only, with the rotational movements of supination and pronation.

The Anatomy of Exercise & Movement

The Elbow Joint

The elbow is a true hinge (ginglymus) joint, meaning it works in only the sagittal plane, and can perform only the actions of flexion and extension. Ligaments and muscles work together to provide stability and mobility to the joint.

The ulnar (medial) collateral ligament is composed of three strong bands, anterior oblique, posterior oblique and transverse, that reinforce the medial side of the articular capsule. The radial (lateral) collateral ligament is a strong triangular ligament that reinforces the lateral side of the articular capsule. These ligaments connect the humerus to the ulna and act together to stabilize the elbow. The annular ligament binds the head of the radius to the ulna, forming the proximal radio-ulnar joint.

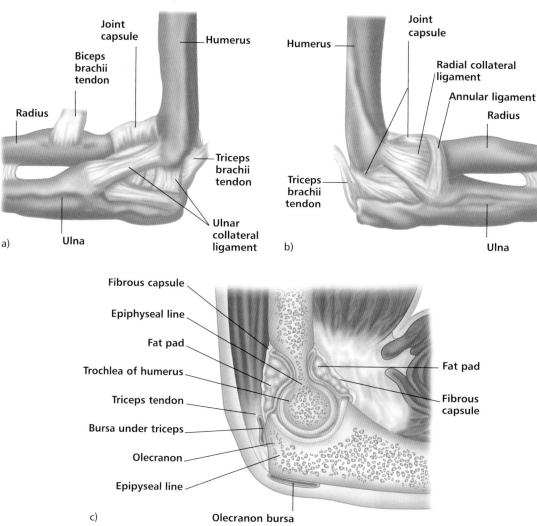

Figure 6.1: The elbow joint (right arm); a) lateral view, b) medial view, c) mid-sagittal view.

The anterior muscles of the elbow are the **biceps brachii**, **brachioradialis**, **brachialis**, and **pronator teres**. The posterior muscles are the **triceps brachii** and the **anconeus**. The tendons of these muscles act as stabilizers, cross the elbow joint, and so provide extra security. It is easy to determine the action of the muscles: the flexors are anterior (anatomical position), the extensors are posterior. Some of the extrinsic muscles in the forearm can also aid flexion, but the contraction is very weak. Terminology helps to decipher some of the muscles:

Biceps = two heads, triceps = three heads.

The biceps brachii translates as two heads and the arm.
The triceps brachii means three heads and the arm.

The biceps and triceps are multi-articulate (working more than one joint), and each have more than one 'head'. This signifies more than two attachment points (usually a muscle has one proximal and one distal tendon attachment to bones).

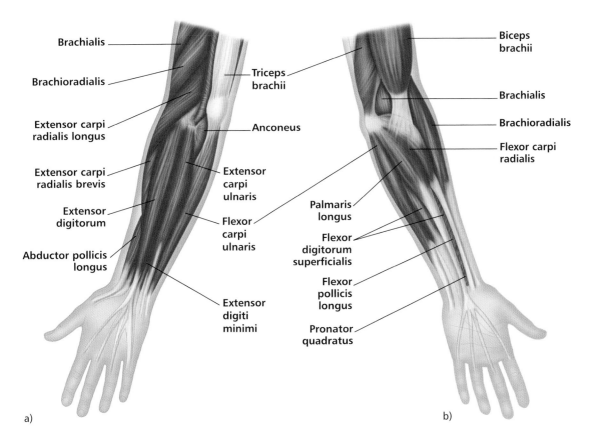

a)   b)

Figure 6.2: Superficial muscles of the arm, a) posterior view, b) anterior view.

Biceps Brachii

Commonly known as the biceps, it passes over three joints: the shoulder, elbow and radio-ulnar, so could be called "tri-articulate". The long and short heads both cross the shoulder joint by proximally attaching to two different parts of the scapula, the coracoid process and glenoid fossa. Both heads come together to form the main muscle belly, which contracts to produce flexion of the shoulder, elbow, and supination of the forearm. Distally, or farther away from the center of the body, the biceps separate again to cross the elbow and insert onto the radius and bicipital aponeurosis.

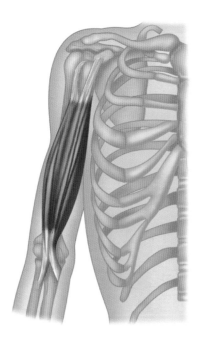
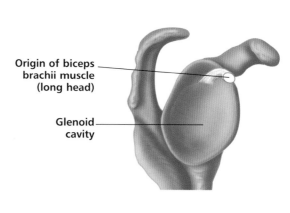

Origin of biceps brachii muscle (long head)

Glenoid cavity

Figure 6.3: Biceps brachii.

Biceps contraction is weak at the shoulder joint; its more important role is stability, maintaining the humeral head in the fossa. It is not a rotator cuff muscle, yet can be affected in the same way if shoulder joint stability is compromised. The long head of the biceps travels through the bicipital groove of the humerus; this small pathway can get cramped, especially if the tendon is inflamed.

Tendonitis is a common over-use injury, and can be healed only by rest and swelling reduction (ice is best, not pills or injections). Any forward movement of the shoulder joint will inhibit the healing process; stretching has been shown to aid in stiff scar tissue build up. Elbow tendonitis is also common (see pages 107–108).

The contraction is stronger at the elbow, where it flexes the joint (the elbow bends). If the forearm is supinated (palm up) as in a biceps curl exercise or chin up, it is even more powerful. When asked to "make a muscle", kids (and adults!) will bend the elbow to show off the biceps. The muscle does not flex, the joint does; a muscle can only contract.

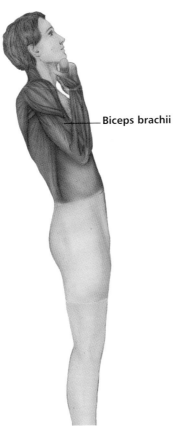

Biceps brachii

Figure 6.4: Chin-ups: the biceps brachii is more powerful when the forearm is supinated (palm up).

Triceps Brachii

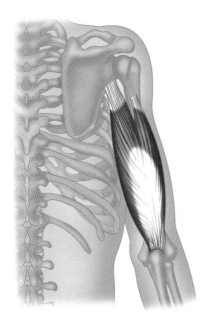

This is one of the few muscles in the human body with three true heads: long, lateral, and medial. The long head is the only one that works the shoulder. It crosses the joint from the humerus to the scapula and extends and adducts the upper arm. The other two heads originate on the upper arm and all three form the muscle belly, then cross the elbow joint to the ulna. It is a biarticulate muscle.

Figure 6.5: Triceps brachii.

At the elbow the triceps is the main extensor, or straightener, of the elbow. Most people think it is the only one, but the small anconeus muscle underneath the triceps helps.

Women tend to have weaker triceps, with a softening of tissue on the underarm as they age. This is directly related to what the arm does daily. In traditional societies, most house work has been done by females; lifting and holding children is also a daily, repetitive movement by many women. These practices are done with the arms in front of the body, therefore working anterior muscles. In fact, most people, no matter what the profession or gender, tend to use the front of the upper body more. The triceps are posterior; the best position to tone the triceps is with the elbow straight and the arm reaching behind the body, using resistance against the reach. One can also push the hand against a wall with the elbow straight, and the triceps will isometrically contract, which strengthens the muscle.

Elbow Strengthening and Stretching Exercises

Many exercises (page numbers indicate those illustrated) can be referred to for strength and stretch of the elbow muscles. Use the following chart for clarification of exercises.

Exercises	Muscles	Strength or Stretch
Biceps curls p.110	Biceps brachii, Brachialis, Brachioradialis	Strength, concentric contraction
Chin-ups, pull-ups p.105/111	Biceps brachii, Brachialis, Brachioradialis	Strength, concentric contraction
Push-ups	Triceps brachii, Anconeus	Strength, concentric contraction
Chataranga dandasana (four-limbed stick pose)	Triceps brachii, Anconeus	Strength, eccentric contraction
Urdhva mukha svanasana (up dog) p.40	Triceps brachii, Anconeus	Strength, concentric contraction
Adho mukha svanasana (down dog) p.40	Triceps brachii, Anconeus	Strength, isometric contraction
Purvottanasana (upward plank pose) p.97	Triceps brachii, Anconeus	Strength, isometric contraction
Dips p.96	Triceps brachii, Anconeus (Biceps brachii at shoulder joint)	Strength, concentric contraction
Elbow stands (dolphin)	Biceps brachii, Brachialis, Brachioradialis	Strength, isometric contraction
Adho mukha vrksasana (handstand) p.119	Triceps brachii, Anconeus	Strength, isometric contraction
Pilates saw p.55	Triceps brachii (front arm) Biceps brachii (back arm)	Stretch
Gomukhasana (cow's face pose)	Triceps brachii (top arm) Biceps brachii (bottom arm)	Stretch
Garudasana (eagle pose) p.111	Triceps brachii (long head)	Stretch
Dhanurasana (bow pose)	Biceps brachii, Brachialis, Brachioradialis	Stretch
Swimming (front stroke)	Biceps brachii and Triceps brachii (depending on part of stroke)	Strength and stretch (depending on part of stroke)
Swimming (back stroke)	Triceps brachii, Anconeus	Strength, concentric contraction (stretch for the biceps)
Rowing	Biceps brachii, Brachialis, Brachioradialis	Strength, concentric contraction
Kayaking	Biceps brachii, Brachialis, Brachioradialis (back arm)	Strength, concentric contraction
	Triceps brachii, Anconeus (front arm)	Strength, concentric contraction

Working the triceps brachii at the elbow joint and the biceps brachii at the shoulder joint:

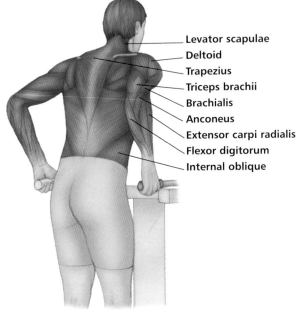

- Levator scapulae
- Deltoid
- Trapezius
- Triceps brachii
- Brachialis
- Anconeus
- Extensor carpi radialis
- Flexor digitorum
- Internal oblique

Figure 6.6: Dips. Triceps brachii and anconeus strength exercise.

TECHNIQUE

Lower body until upper arms are parallel to the floor. Knees should be slightly behind hips and chest slightly in front. Return to the starting position by extending elbows.

Elbow Injuries

Tennis Elbow (Lateral Epicondylitis)

Both the lateral and medial sides of the elbow are insertion points for tendons that also direct wrist and hand movements. This common tendon attachment can become inflamed, particularly with repetitive movements involving gripping and twisting, such as in playing tennis, or turning a screwdriver. Gardening can also be a culprit. There is usually tenderness to the lateral elbow, and with acute injuries some swelling can be present. This is a tendonitis issue, and therefore rest and reduction of inflammation is necessary. Physical therapy might be helpful; prevention is to manage any muscle tightness or weaknesses.

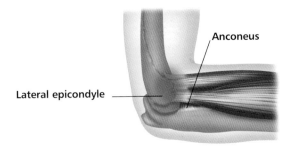

Anconeus

Lateral epicondyle

Figure 6.7: Tennis elbow.

Golfers' Elbow (Medial Epicondylitis)

Golfers' elbow is less common, but similar, to tennis elbow, where the common tendon attachment on the inside of the joint can become inflamed. This happens with repetitive movements involving gripping and carrying loads, or when a medial force is directed upward, as in a golf swing. Proper technique, and stretching after a game may help to prevent this condition.

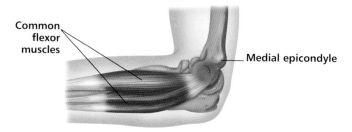

Figure 6.8: Golfers' elbow.

The Radio-ulnar Joint

Supination is best described at this joint as the palm facing forward (anatomical position), also called 'palm up'. The radius externally rotates to a parallel position with the ulna. In **pronation**, the palm of the hand faces backward, or 'palm down'. The radius rotates internally so that it lies diagonally across the ulna.

The radius and ulna join at two different articulation points: proximal and distal. The bones are curved, otherwise they would hit each other as the radius rotates. At the proximal end (near the elbow), there is a 'ring' formed by the radial notch and the annular ligament, lined with synovial membrane. This ring allows easier rotation of the radius during pronation. At the distal end (near the wrist) there is an articular disc that is a strong attachment point for the ulna and radius. The interosseous membrane also connects the two bones and limits excess supination.

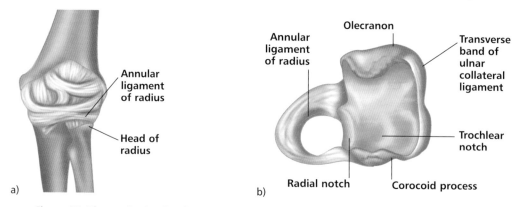

Figure 6.9: The proximal radio-ulnar joint, a) left arm, anterior view, b) left arm, superior view.

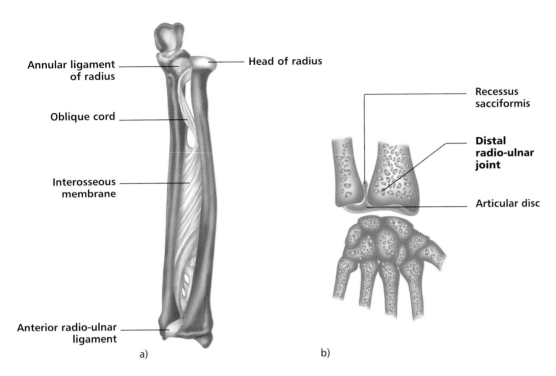

Figure 6.10: The distal radio-ulnar joint, a) left arm, anterior view, b) left arm/hand, coronal view.

These movements are necessary for many everyday activities: turning a key or screwdriver, turning pages, holding an object up in the palm of the hand. If these movements occur with the elbow straight, they can be confused with shoulder joint rotation. Pronation at the radio-ulnar joint can accompany internal shoulder rotation; extreme supination can allow shoulder external rotation. Flex the elbow and one can easily see how the joint moves by itself.

Muscles of the Radio-ulnar Joint

The two main pronators are the **pronator teres** and **pronator quadratus**. The teres is proximal, crossing the elbow to assist in flexion. The quadratus is distal, and pulls the radius across the ulna.

The two primary supinators are the **biceps brachii** and the **supinator** muscles. The biceps help uncross the upper radius from a pronated position. The supinator has two layers and wraps around the radius to allow supination. It can be isolated from the biceps by extending the elbow while supinating, as in a baseball pitch with a curve. When the elbow is flexed the biceps are engaged more in supination, such as the biceps curl exercise.

A fifth muscle comes into play in both actions: the **brachioradialis**. It is mainly an elbow flexor, but from extreme pronation can supinate back to neutral, and from extreme supination, can pronate back to neutral. It can be seen on most individuals as a prominent forearm muscle.

The Anatomy of Exercise & Movement

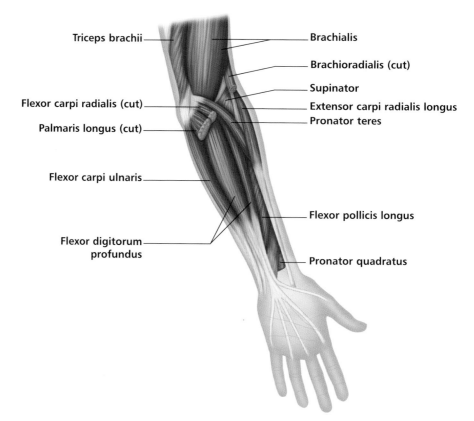

Triceps brachii

Brachialis

Brachioradialis (cut)

Supinator

Flexor carpi radialis (cut)

Extensor carpi radialis longus

Palmaris longus (cut)

Pronator teres

Flexor carpi ulnaris

Flexor pollicis longus

Flexor digitorum profundus

Pronator quadratus

Figure 6.11: Deep muscles of the arm (anterior view).

Radio-ulnar Joint Exercises

Hand weights and dumbbells are useful in developing this joint. While doing an elbow curl, simply supinate as the elbow flexes, and pronate as it extends. One can also do this with pulleys, or it can be incorporated into the Pilates 100.

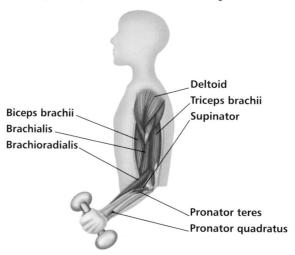

Deltoid

Triceps brachii

Supinator

Biceps brachii

Brachialis

Brachioradialis

Pronator teres

Pronator quadratus

Figure 6.12: Biceps curl using dumbbell to strengthen elbow joint.

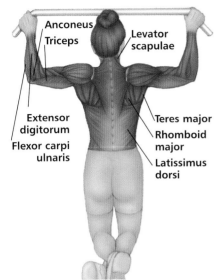

Anconeus
Triceps
Levator scapulae
Extensor digitorum
Flexor carpi ulnaris
Teres major
Rhomboid major
Latissimus dorsi

The overhand grip on a bar or dumbbell is indicated for pronation, with thumbs facing each other. An upright row exercise uses this grip. If hanging from a bar in the pronated position it would be called a 'pull-up', as the body raises.

The underhand grip is a supinated position, where thumbs are outward from each other. This happens in a chin-up, where the biceps brachii would be concentrically contracting on the way up, and eccentrically contracting on the way down (see figure 6.4).

Figure 6.13: Pull-ups.

TECHNIQUE

With palms facing away from the body on a high bar at least shoulder-width apart, begin to pull the body up, then lower; repetitions and sets can be used to overload, therefore strengthen the muscles.

In Yoga, most postures are done in a pronated position. Arm balances will actually affect the wrist more. One can always supinate and pronate while doing **Warrior II**.

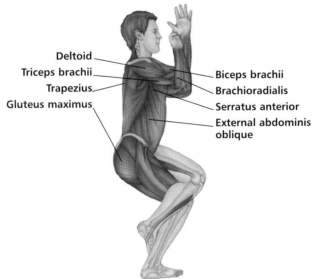

Deltoid
Triceps brachii
Trapezius
Gluteus maximus
Biceps brachii
Brachioradialis
Serratus anterior
External abdominis oblique

Figure 6.14: Garudasana (eagle pose).

TECHNIQUE

Cross the right arm over the left at the elbows, then supinate (turn the palms toward each other) as the elbows bend. Hold for the stretch; repeat on the other side. The full pose also involves standing on one leg and wrapping the opposite foot around it as the knees and hips flex. The forearms will easily pronate; adding supination will deepen the pose and complete the asana.

Myths of the Elbow and Radio-ulnar Joints Dispelled

The elbow does not rotate

The elbow is a true hinge joint, which means it can only work in the sagittal plane and do the actions of flexion and extension. This happens primarily at the articulation point of the humerus and ulna. Rotation in the transverse, or horizontal plane, happens at a separate joint, the radio-ulnar joint, below the elbow. **Rotation of the forearm (supination and pronation) occurs at the junction of the radius and ulna bones, not the elbow. This allows the hand to turn up or down.**

'Tennis' and 'golf elbow' are not just from sports

Two common injuries at the elbow are overuse injuries: tennis elbow and golfer's elbow. Golfer's elbow involves the tendon of the common flexor, which originates at the medial epicondyle of the humerus on the inside of the elbow. Tennis elbow is a similar injury, but at the common extensor origin on the outside of the elbow, the lateral epicondyle of the humerus. Both injuries are actually tendonitis, which can also happen in other activities such as excessive gardening and house-cleaning. **Extreme repetition can cause injury.**

The angle of the elbow bones are not straight

There is an odd alignment when the arm is straight (extended), with the palm facing forward or up (supination), called the 'carrying angle'. The bones of the humerus and forearm are not perfectly aligned. There is a deviation from a straight line that occurs in the direction of the thumb, noticeable in anatomical position. This angle permits the arm to be swung without hitting the hips. It can vary, especially between the dominant and non-dominant hand. **"Form follows function". Natural forces can affect body position.**

Main Muscles Involved in Movements of the Elbow and Radio-ulnar Joints

Elbow Joint

Flexion
Brachialis; Biceps Brachii; Brachioradialis; Pronator Teres; Extensor Carpi Radialis Longus and Brevis; Flexor Carpi Radialis and Ulnaris; Flexor Digitorum Superficialis; Palmaris Longus (the last 6 muscles are weak elbow flexors)

Extension
Triceps Brachii; Anconeus; Extensor Carpi Ulnaris; Extensor Digitorum & Minimi are weak extensors

Radio-ulnar Joint

Supination
Supinator; Biceps Brachii; Brachioradialis; Extensor Pollicis Longus; Extensor Indicis & Abductor Pollicis Longus are weak supinators

Pronation
Pronator Quadratus; Pronator Teres; Brachioradialis; Flexor Carpi Radialis, Extensor Carpi Radialis Brevis are weak pronators

Chapter

7

The Wrist and Hand

The wrist and hand together are made up of twenty-seven bones, numerous ligaments, and many muscles and tendons, which provide for fine motor capabilities of the fingers. The wrist and palm house the eight carpal bones, whose proximal row, comprising the scaphoid, lunate, triquetrum and pisiform, articulates with the radius and ulna to create the radiol-carpal joint. This is where the main actions of the wrist take place; as a condyloid (ellipsoid) joint, it can do flexion, extension, abduction and adduction. The combination of these four actions is circumduction.

The Anatomy of Exercise & Movement

The distal row of the carpals, comprising trapezium, trapezoid, capitate and hamate, meets the five metacarpals, which articulate with the proximal phalanges. Each finger has three phalanges, whereas the thumb only has two. This metacarpo-phalangeal joint is also a condyloid joint. The interphalangeal joints are hinge joints, where flexion and extension of the fingers occur.

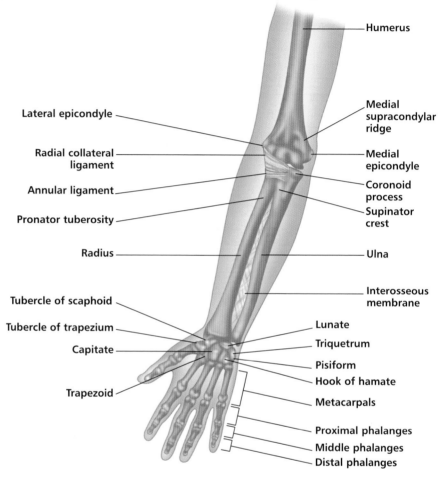

Figure 7.1: The bones of the right forearm and hand (anterior view).

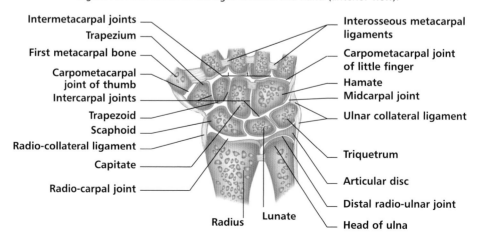

Figure 7.2: The radio-carpal (wrist), intercarpal, carpometacarpal and intermetacarpal joints (coronal view).

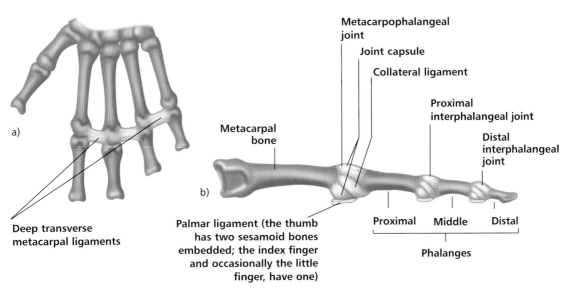

Figure 7.3: The metacarpophalangeal and interphalangeal joints; a) anterior view, b) medial view.

The human hand is a wondrous device of dexterity. It has many small joints, with the most significant being the saddle joint of the thumb. This is where the action of 'opposition' takes place, allowing the thumb to touch each finger separately.

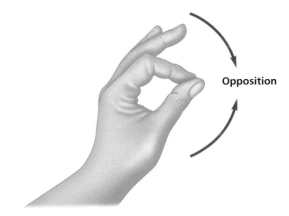

Figure 7.4: Opposition takes place at the saddle joint of the thumb, allowing the thumb to touch each finger of the same hand separately.

Without this action people would not have evolved to this technological age. The specialization of the human hand has made us able to build fires, make tools, and shape the world. The action of opposition sets humans apart from other primates. The muscles that do this are in the palm of the hand.

Ligaments of the Wrist and Hand

With so many bones to hold together, the ligaments of the wrist and hand are numerous. Main ones to be aware of are the following:

1. Flexor retinaculum is a wide ligament that crosses the carpals horizontally on the palmar side of the hand. It connects the hamate and pisiform to the scaphoid and trapezium, which ensures stability of the carpals. This ligament helps form the narrow space called the carpal tunnel, where the tendons of many flexors of the hand pass through.

2. Extensor retinaculum is a posterior, or dorsal ligament that attaches to the radius, then across to the ulna, triquetrum, and pisiform. It holds the extensor tendons in place.

3. Interosseous carpal ligaments connect the lunate to the scaphoid and triquetrum, and help stabilize the wrist joint cavity.

4. Interosseous and deep transverse metacarpal ligaments are the inter-metacarpal ligaments and help support the structure of the palm of the hand.

5. Medial and lateral collateral ligaments on the sides of the carpals support the hand by attaching the ulna to the fifth phalange on the medial side, and the radius to the thumb on the lateral side. There are also collateral ligaments that help hold the metacarpophalangeal joints together.

6. Palmar ligament is a dense band of fibro-cartilaginous tissue that reinforces the metacarpophalangeal joints on the palmar side of the hand.

There is also an important connective tissue structure called the **palmar aponeurosis**, which extends from the flexor retinaculum to the four fingers and is attached to the skin of the palm. This 'compartment' helps keep the tendons in place.

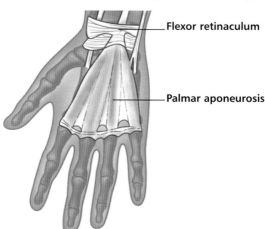

Flexor retinaculum

Palmar aponeurosis

Figure 7.5: Example of wrist/hand ligament, flexor retinaculum, and the connective tissue, palmar aponeurosis.

Muscles of the Wrist

Main movers of the wrist seem complicated, but their nomenclature makes it easy:

- If the muscle flexes the wrist, 'flexor' is used in the name of the muscle.
- If it abducts (indicating wrist movement to the outside, or lateral side in anatomical position) the term 'radialis' is included, meaning toward the radial (thumb) side.
- If the muscle extends the wrist, the term 'extensor' is used in the name.
- If it adducts (indicating medial movement toward the body from anatomical position) the term 'ulnaris', or 'toward the pinky side', is used.
- Other muscles that work the thumb are indicated by the word 'pollicis'.

Therefore, the following muscles are named in accordance with the joint actions they create:

Flexor carpi radialis (flexion and abduction); **flexor carpi ulnaris** (flexion and adduction); **extensor carpi radialis longus** (extension and abduction); **extensor carpi radialis brevis** (extension and abduction); **extensor carpi ulnaris** (extension and adduction). The wrist flexors are located anteriorly, and the extensors posteriorly (see figure 6.2 & 6.11).

Injuries/Conditions of the Wrist and Hand

The fine motor skills of the hand allow us to grasp, reach, hold, write, touch; in short, communicate. The muscles are supplied by the **brachial plexus**, a group of spinal nerves (cervical nerves 5 through 8 and the thoracic nerve) that supply motor and sensory function to the upper extremity. The ulnar, radial, and median nerves are extended from this system and innervate the muscles of the wrist and hand. This is important because of two conditions that are common: **carpel tunnel syndrome** and **numbness in the fingers**.

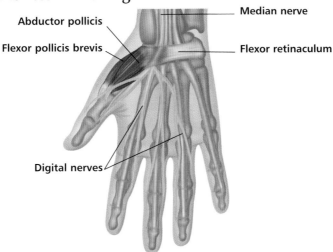

Figure 7.6: Carpal tunnel syndrome.

The median nerve travels through the carpal bones of the wrist joint. There is an area, or tunnel, that the nerve and flexor tendons share. Pressure in this carpal tunnel can increase when tendons are inflamed, interfering with normal function of the median nerve. This is what is known as **carpal tunnel syndrome**, a painfully chronic condition brought on by overuse of the wrist joint in activities such as typing and cleaning.

Surgery is performed to relieve the pain of this injury; unfortunately too many surgeries. There are new movement techniques being developed by professionals that hopefully will bypass surgery and ease this condition. A physical therapist can help stretch and strengthen this smaller area of movement, where the carpal bones tend to glide instead of completing true joint movements.

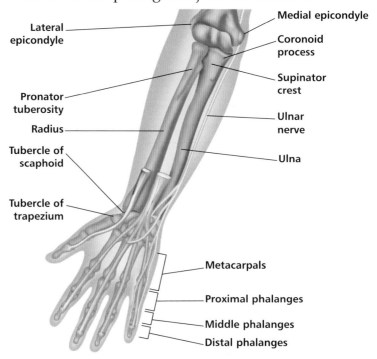

Figure 7.7: Ulnar tunnel syndrome (anterior view).

A similar condition, **ulnar tunnel syndrome**, can result in pain, loss of sensation and muscle weakness in the hand. The ulnar nerve runs along the inside of the forearm, reaching down to the heel of the hand, where it radiates across the palm and into the little finger and ring finger.

PREVENTION

Prevention is important. If the wrist is hyperextended, the flexors of the wrist will stretch and the carpal area will 'open up'. Place the palms on the floor with fingers facing the body while kneeling or sitting. This can also be done standing with the palm on a wall and fingers facing out. The stretch should be done before inflammation sets in.

Working at computer or piano keyboards for hours can create stress in the wrists and hands. There are a few different modalities that can aid this. Hand drumming is an excellent way to exercise the hands in a different way. Yoga also has some important hand balances that can help. The **down dog** and **handstand** are two very efficient wrist strengtheners, if done the correct way. The wrist is hyperextended, the fingers are extended; this can create tension or even pain unless the weight is on the ball of the hand, specifically under the thumb and forefinger, allowing pressure on the palm to be relieved.

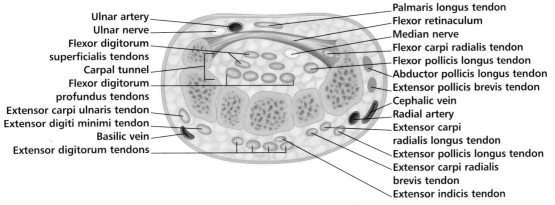

Figure 7.8: Cross-section of the wrist.

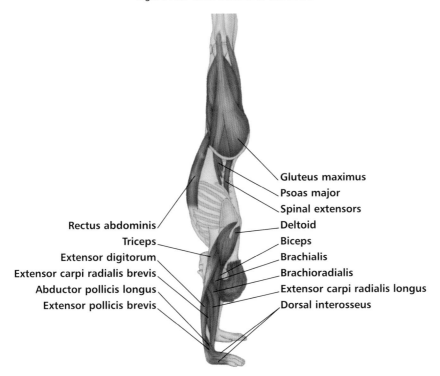

Figure 7.9: Adho mukha vrksasana (handstand).

Numbness of the fingers can be related to pinched nerves in the brachial plexus originating from the cervical and thoracic areas of the spine. Nerves can be affected by trauma, tight or spasmodic muscles, bone misalignment, or bulging discs (the cartilage between the vertebrae, not the bone itself.) Correct alignment and exercises to alleviate pinched nerves are found in Chapter 3. **Prevention is correct posture.**

The Anatomy of Exercise & Movement

Wrist and Hand Stretching Exercises

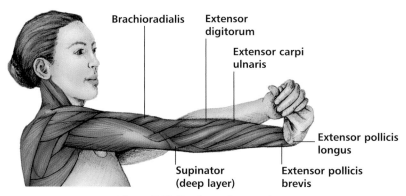

Figure 7.10: Turning wrist stretch.

TECHNIQUE

Place one arm straight out in front and parallel to the ground. Turn the wrist down and outward and then use the other hand to further turn the hand upward.

Stretches for the Brachial Plexus

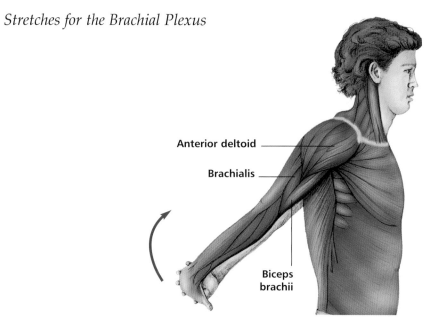

Figure 7.11: Behind the back chest stretch.

TECHNIQUE

Reach/clasp hands behind the back and raise arms with the back straight. Circle the arm backward (circumduction).

TECHNIQUE

Move the arm through its ranges of motion while stretching the head away from it.

Myths of the Wrist and Hand Dispelled

The wrist and fingers do not rotate
It might 'look' like they do, but what is happening is not rotation, it is circumduction. This can happen at any condyloid joint, and is a combination of flexion, extension, abduction and adduction. **Any appearance of rotary movement in the forearm to the hand is caused by pronation and supination at the radio-ulnar joint, which is not the wrist joint or hand.**

The wrist and hand are complicated, yet fragile
The anatomical design of both the wrist and hand is remarkable. This design allows humans to be different from any other primate. As wonderful as it is, its susceptibility to injury is common. Any time someone falls, the hand reaches out to break the impact to the body. This is a natural, neuromuscular response, and one that can lead to sprains, strains, and fractures of the area. **Exercises can be done to strengthen the wrist and hand, and can be incorporated into any workout.**

The carpal area can be unstable
The eight carpal bones can glide, which means they have a little 'give' to them as the palm of the hand is used. With the advent of more people in many sports, athletes are experiencing an increase in injuries to this area, as well as keyboard operators (computers!). More research is needed on how to condition the area, as it is hard to prevent injury here; the tube that the median nerve passes through is narrow and tissue can get irritated, mostly by overuse when the wrist is flexed. **The hands are unique. We should take better care of them.**

Main Muscles Involved in Movements of the Wrist, Hand, Fingers and Thumb

Radio-carpal and Midcarpal Joints

Flexion
Flexor Carpi Radialis; Flexor Carpi Ulnaris; Palmaris Longus; Flexor Digitorum Superficialis; Flexor Digitorum Profundus; Flexor Pollicis Longus; Abductor Pollicis Longus; Extensor Pollicis Brevis

Extension
Extensor Carpi Radialis Brevis; Extensor Carpi Radialis Longus; Extensor Carpi Ulnaris; Extensor Digitorum; Extensor Indicis; Extensor Pollicis Longus; Extensor Digiti Minimi

Abduction
Extensor Carpi Radialis Brevis; Extensor Carpi Radialis Longus; Flexor Carpi Radialis; Abductor Pollicis Longus; Extensor Pollicis Longus; Extensor Pollicis Brevis

Adduction
Flexor Carpi Ulnaris; Extensor Carpi Ulnaris

Metacarpophalangeal Joints of the Fingers

Flexion
Flexor Digitorum Profundus; Flexor Digitorum Superficialis; Lumbricales; Interossei; Flexor Digiti Minimi; Abductor Digiti Minimi; Palmaris Longus (through palmar aponeurosis)

Extension
Extensor Digitorum; Extensor Indicis; Extensor Digiti Minimi

Abduction and Adduction
Interossei; Abductor Digiti Minimi; Lumbricales (may assist in radial deviation); Extensor Digitorum (abducts by hyperextending; tendon to index radially deviates); Flexor Digitorum Profundus (adducts by flexing); Flexor Digitorum Superficialis (adducts by flexing)

Rotation
Lumbricales; Interossei (movement slight except index; only effective when phalanx is flexed); Opponens Digiti Minimi (rotates little finger at carpometacarpal joint)

Interphalangeal Joints of the Fingers

Flexion
Flexor Digitorum Profundus (both joints); Flexor Digitorum Superficialis (proximal joint only)

Extension
Extensor Digitorum; Extensor Digiti Minimi; Extensor Indicis; Lumbricales; Interossei

Carpometacarpal Joint of the Thumb

Flexion
Flexor Pollicis Brevis; Flexor Pollicis Longus; Opponens Pollicis

Extension
Extensor Pollicis Brevis; Extensor Pollicis Longus; Abductor Pollicis Longus

Abduction
Abductor Pollicis Brevis; Abductor Pollicis Longus

Adduction
Adductor Pollicis; Dorsal Interossei (first only); Extensor Pollicis Longus (in full extension/abduction); Flexor Pollicis Longus (in full extension/abduction)

Opposition
Opponens Pollicis; Abductor Pollicis Brevis; Flexor Pollicis Brevis; Flexor Pollicis Longus; Adductor Pollicis

Metacarpophalangeal Joint of the Thumb

Flexion
Flexor Pollicis Brevis; Flexor Pollicis Longus; Palmar Interossei (first only); Abductor Pollicis Brevis

Extension
Extensor Pollicis Brevis; Extensor Pollicis Longus

Abduction
Abductor Pollicis Brevis

Adduction
Adductor Pollicis; Palmar Interossei (first only)

Interphalangeal Joint of the Thumb

Flexion
Flexor Pollicis Longus

Extension
Abductor Pollicis Brevis; Extensor Pollicis Longus; Adductor Pollicis; Extensor Pollicis Brevis (occasional insertion)

Chapter

8

The Iliofemoral (Hip) Joint

The iliofemoral joint is a large ball-and-socket joint formed by the articulation between the acetabulum of the pelvis (the socket) and the head of the femur (the ball). In architectural concepts, the pelvis is the keystone and the femurs are the flying buttresses of an arch-like shape. This structure makes the hip joint very stable.

The muscles that work the hip pass from the pelvis to the femur, some even going past the knee joint. All the larger muscles shape the thigh. Muscles on the front of the thigh flex the hip, the outside (lateral) muscles abduct, the back thigh muscles extend, and the inside (medial) adduct. Most of the above also perform inward or outward rotation, the final two actions of the hip.

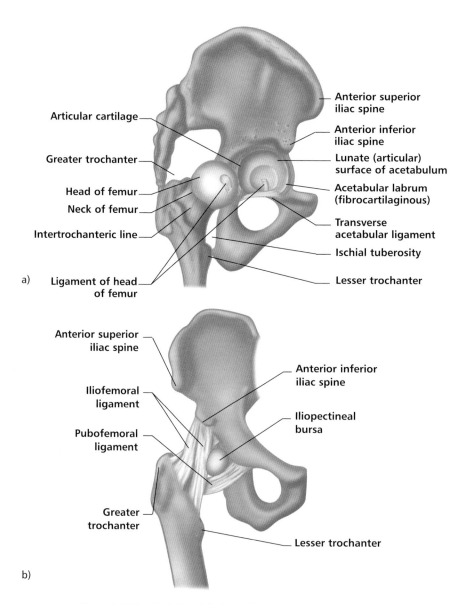

Figure 8.1: The hip joint, right leg, a) lateral view, b) anterior view.

Anterior Hip (Flexor) Muscles

Primary movers of flexion: **rectus femoris, sartorius, iliopsoas.**

The **rectus femoris** is the most superficial flexor of the thigh. It is also a member of the quadriceps muscle group, extending the knee. Because it works two joints, it is termed '**biarticulate**'. It is the only large muscle of the hip that can do only one action at the hip. It can allow a forward tilt of the pelvis when it is short, or tight; weak abdominal muscles are also responsible for this postural misalignment. Because of its actions at the hip and knee, it is a powerful running muscle.

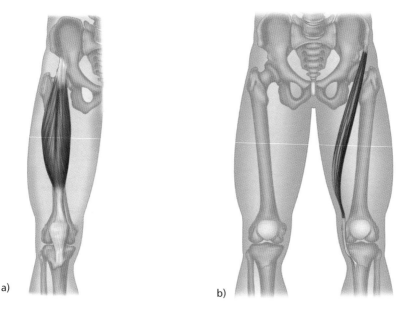

Figure 8.2: a) Rectus femoris, and b) sartorius.

The **sartorius** is the longest muscle in the human body, crossing the hip joint from the lateral, or outside of the pelvis, diagonally down to the medial, or inside, of the knee. When the hip is flexed, it is also an outward rotator. When contracted it can tilt the pelvis forward, similar to the rectus femoris; the abdominals are needed to counteract this movement. The sartorius is especially active in forward soccer kicks that outward rotate the hip and extend the knee, and in ballet battements to the front and side.

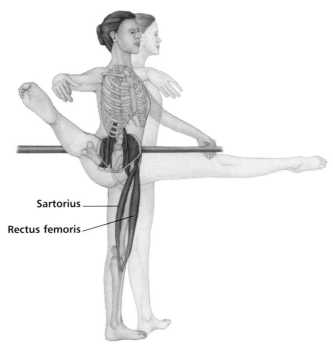

Sartorius ———

Rectus femoris ———

Figure 8.3: a) Ballet front battements (ghost effect), b) side battements.
(The rectus femoris is working in hip flexion and knee extension,
while the sartorius is flexing and externally rotating the hip.)

The **iliopsoas** muscle group is the deepest of the hip flexors. These muscles are the **iliacus**, the **psoas major**, and the **psoas minor**. Detailed information on this muscle group can be found in Chapter 4.

Like the first two flexors, if tight it can contribute to anterior pelvic tilt, creating too much forward curve in the lumbar area. This is a common condition in young dancers. It can be alleviated by stretching properly, not forcing turnout, and being more aware of the **working center** (abdominals, pelvis, and lower spine).

The iliopsoas is in strong contraction when doing a sit-up with straight legs (the **Pilates roll-up**) but the abdominals also need to be strong to prevent the lower back from being aggravated. If sit-ups are done with bent knees (hips are already flexed), the iliopsoas will work less as the abdominals flex the spine.

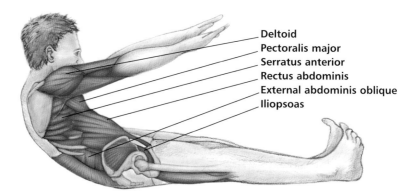

Deltoid
Pectoralis major
Serratus anterior
Rectus abdominis
External abdominis oblique
Iliopsoas

Figure 8.4: Pilates roll-up.

TECHNIQUE

Lying supine, extend legs together and dorsiflex the feet. Reach the arms to the ceiling and inhale; on the exhale, roll the head off the floor and slowly continue to roll up the spine, deepening the abdominals and reaching for the toes. Keep heels on the floor – if that is impossible, bend the knees or use the hands against the floor while maintaining the integrity of the exercise.

Roll downs are just as effective, if not more so. Not because they are harder to do; they are actually easier due to gravity helping. Rolling back down to the floor from a straight sitting position, the abdominals and psoas work eccentrically as each spinal area articulates into the floor (keep the chin toward the chest and go slow). During the roll-up or roll down, secondary hip flexors are the **pectineus** and **tensor fasciae latae** muscles. They are described in more detail later.

Hip Flexor Strengthening Exercises

All walking, running, jumping, leaping, hopping, and kicking movements will work the hip flexors in some way, whether as agonists, antagonists, or stabilizers. This is dependent on the phase of the movement. **Agonists** are the main muscle movers of a particular joint action. **Antagonists** are usually located opposite the main movers, counteracting the action. **Stabilizers**, also called **fixators**, are muscles acting as a firm base while other muscles exert force to create movement.

All skeletal muscles are movers and stabilizers – it depends on the movement and position of the body as to how the muscles are reacting at the time. Skeletal muscles are all of the above – it depends on the movement and position of the body as to what role the muscles are playing at the time.

Cardiovascular machines are great hip joint workouts in the sagittal plane, which means the joint actions of flexion and extension are being done. The treadmill is especially good; walking or running outdoors is even better (fresh air!) as long as proper footwear and running surfaces are available.

1. Supine Hip Flexion (Level I)

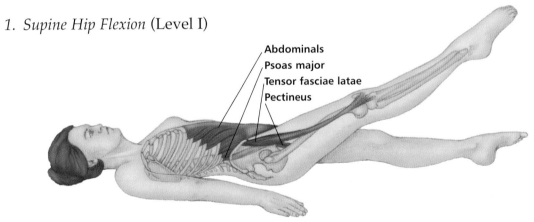

Abbreviations in figure:
Abdominals
Psoas major
Tensor fasciae latae
Pectineus

Figure 8.5: Supine hip flexion (level I).

TECHNIQUE

Lie on back and raise one leg to a 45-degree angle. Keeping the knee bent will be easier, straight is harder. Engage the abdominals, holding the position for at least 10 seconds. Add ankle weights if needed for more resistance. Repeat on the other leg. Do not raise both legs at the same time! There is much evidence that shows the lower back is too compromised in this position, as the psoas major is working overtime because of its origin on the lower back and insertion on the femur.

In a ballet 'floor barre' class, one would lie supine and lift one leg up to 90 degrees or higher (toward ceiling). Lift and lower slowly while gravity resists. Repeat 8–10 times on each leg. Include hip rotation for added muscle work. This can also be done standing at the barre (see figure 8.3), and will feel more difficult due to gravity and the lack of floor support.

Many standing Yoga postures will work the hip flexors because the thigh is in front of the hip, usually in isometric contraction. Warrior poses (**virabhadrasanas**) are especially good, as the front knee bends over the toe (not beyond), and the thigh is held in parallel or in a slightly turned out position. It is the front leg flexors that are being strengthened.

2. Standing Yoga Postures (Levels I–III)

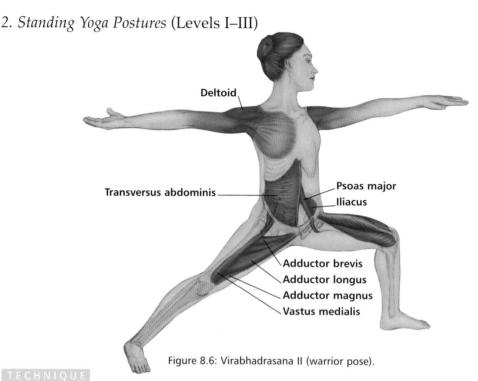

Figure 8.6: Virabhadrasana II (warrior pose).

TECHNIQUE

From a standing position (tadasana, mountain pose), step back with left leg 3-4 feet; the front foot remains forward while the back toes turn in (approx. 30-60 degrees). Bend the front knee over the toes as the back leg remains straight. Hips will open as weight is centered between both legs and arms stretch out to the sides. Hold for at least 30 seconds before doing the other side. Warrior I, III, and triangle pose are also good for flexors.

A Note About Squats

Squats are one of the most popular exercises in the weight room. Many students are convinced that squats work the hip flexors. The only hip flexor worked in a squat is the rectus femoris, and that is because it is a quadriceps muscle that extends the knee. Keep in mind that the most important part of the squat is on the way up from a sitting position, against gravity and weight. The knees are extending (quadriceps) and the hips are extending (gluteus maximus and hamstrings) in concentric contraction. On the way down these same muscles are eccentrically contracting, to keep the body from collapsing to the floor. Therefore, **the hip flexors as a whole are not the main movers in any part of the squat exercise**. The same principle applies for the plié in dance.

A Note About Pilates

Pilates mat work incorporates a lot of hip flexion. Many exercises are done sitting or lying down with the legs in the air. This is not a problem if the abdominals are truly engaged to counteract the pull of the hip flexors and weight of the femur (the heaviest bone in the body).

To offset hip flexion positions in Pilates, the following prone exercises can be done:

1. Swan prep
2. Swan dive

3. Single/double leg kicks
4. Swim

These are usually introduced toward the middle of a full routine. In a beginning Pilates mat class one can always incorporate more stretches for the hip flexors to 'open up' the front of the hip. Once a student has grasped the concept of the correct use of the abdominals as stabilizers, hip flexion should not be a problem.

Sitting is hip flexion. Everyone needs to stretch the hip flexors to keep them from shortening in **too much sitting**!

Hip Flexor Stretching Exercises

Any exercise that stretches the abdominals will also stretch the hip flexors, as demonstrated in Chapter 4.

1. Setu Bandha (Bridge) (Level I)

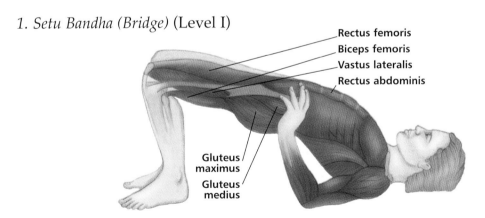

Figure 8.7: Setu bandha (bridge pose) (level I). (Not visible: sartorius, iliopsoas.)

TECHNIQUE

Lie on back with knees bent, hands by sides or underneath tailbone, feet flat on floor 6–8 inches apart. Lift hips off floor and push toward ceiling, allowing weight to rest on shoulders and feet. Hold for up to one minute, breathing deeply. On an exhale, roll back down through the spine.

The Anatomy of Exercise & Movement

2. *Posterior Leg Lifts* (Level I)

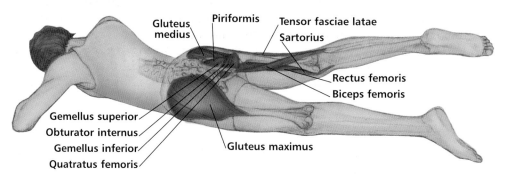

Figure 8.8: Posterior leg lifts (level I).

TECHNIQUE

Lie prone (on stomach), resting forehead on hands. Lift right leg a few inches off floor, with right hip still connected to floor. Extend the leg out from the hip joint. Increase the stretch by bending the knee, foot toward the ceiling – if there are no knee problems, hold the ankle.

3. *Lunges* (Level II)

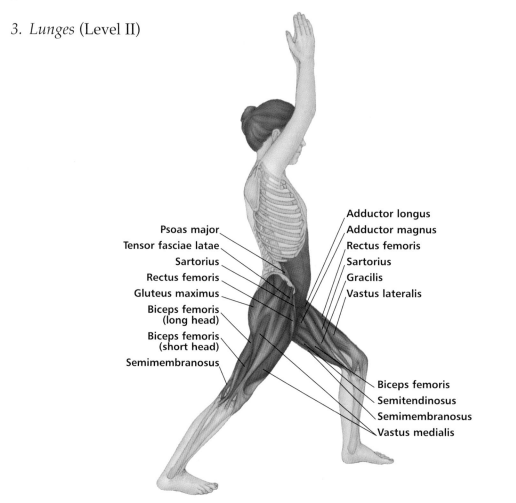

Figure 8.9: Virabhadrasana I (warrior pose). In lunges, the legs are positioned the same way, sometimes deeper, as in a runner's stretch described under technique.

TECHNIQUE

Begin standing with left foot forward, right leg back. Bend the front knee until it is directly over toes; slide right leg straight back until parallel to the floor, if possible. Keep feet facing forward and do not let front knee go farther than toes. The spine is straight and hands can rest on front thigh, or raise up. **The hip flexors are strengthening in the front leg, stretching in the back leg.** Hold for approximately 30 seconds, then repeat on the other side. Warrior poses in Yoga **(virabhadrasanas I, II, and III)** are similar; **warrior I** is pictured.

4. *Ustrasana (Camel Pose)* (Level II–III)

TECHNIQUE

This is a backbend that opens the chest and shoulders, as well as stretching the hip flexors and abdominals. Kneel (both knees can be on a blanket for comfort) with knees and feet in line parallel with each other, and the upper body completely straight, hands on hips or sacral area for support. Begin to arch back, bending the thoracic area while extending the head and lifting the sternum. Allow the shoulder-blades to come together and down the spine while the abdominals lift.

5. *The Pilates Swan Dive* (Level III)

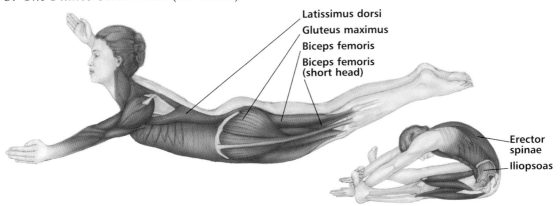

Latissimus dorsi
Gluteus maximus
Biceps femoris
Biceps femoris (short head)

Erector spinae
Iliopsoas

Figure 8.10: The Pilates swan dive (level III), and then afterward stretch forward (inset).

TECHNIQUE

Lie prone with heels together, adding a forward and backward rock. One must have a very strong back for this exercise. Afterward stretch the back and hips.

Lateral Hip (Abductor) Muscles

Primary movers of abduction: **tensor fasciae latae, gluteus medius, gluteus minimus.**

The **tensor fasciae latae** is found on the outside of the thigh, crossing the hip joint from the iliac crest into the **ilio-tibial band (ITB)**. This band, or tract, is a combination of two muscles, the gluteus maximus and the tensor fasciae latae, plus fascia (connective tissue). It extends down past the outside of the knee to the tibia and is important in stabilizing the hip and knee in standing and walking.

The Anatomy of Exercise & Movement

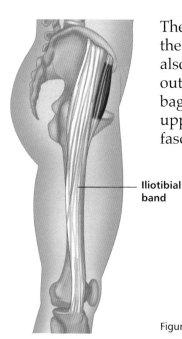

The main action of the tensor fasciae latae is abduction of the hip; when the thigh is flexed and inward rotated it is also quite active. It is not a strong flexor when the hip is outward rotated. People who complain about 'saddle bags' (which can be described as a protuberance on the upper outside of the thigh) have located the tensor fasciae latae muscle and need to tone it.

Iliotibial band

Figure 8.11: Tensor fasciae latae.

The **gluteus medius** lies directly under the maximus, with a small portion of it appearing above, or superior, attaching all the way up toward the iliac crest of the pelvis. People who have posterior 'high hips' could have a well-developed gluteus medius – the top portion can be seen easily. The medius then crosses the ilio-femoral joint to attach distally to the femur's greater trochanter, allowing the muscle to work the hip joint.

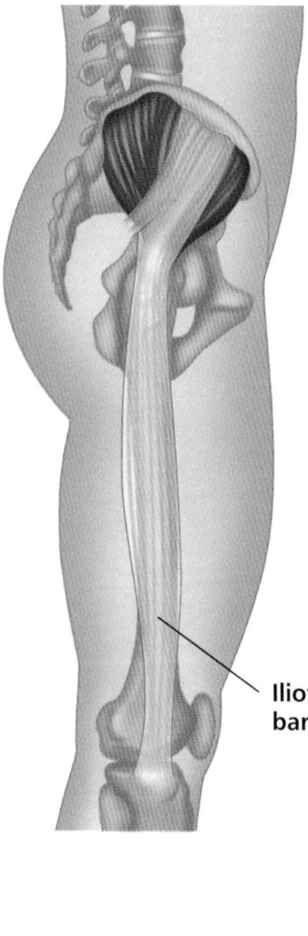

A common myth is that the gluteus muscles all work together, or are **complete synergists** (performing all the same actions); this is not always true of the maximus in relation to the other two glutei. The anterior gluteus medius is responsible for two major hip actions that the gluteus maximus cannot do well: abduction and medial rotation (only the anterior, superior fibers of the gluteus maximus might abduct, and this is minimal). Hip abduction is the action of the thigh going away from the center of the body in the frontal plane, with the leg moving 'out to the side'.

Iliotibial band

Figure 8.12: Gluteus medius and the iliotibial band (ITB).

In medial, or inward or internal rotation, the head of the femur rolls in toward the body. If the feet are 'pigeon-toed', the hips are usually inward rotated. Only the front, or anterior, fibers of the gluteus medius can inwardly rotate. The posterior fibers actually outwardly rotate as the leg abducts, making it more synergistic with the anterior, superior fibers of the gluteus maximus. Muscles are complicated.

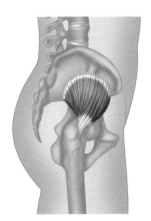

The deepest glute, the **minimus**, is also the smallest. It is slightly anterior and synergistic with the anterior portion of the gluteus medius, as well as the tensor fasciae latae. This means it abducts and inward rotates the hip. It can aid in flexion, but only as a weaker mover. All abduction exercises will also work the gluteus minimus.

Figure 8.13: Gluteus minimus.

When the pelvis tilts forward, the gluteus minimus is active, if the femur is fixed. The minimus can work during all phases of pelvic mobility.

Hip Abductor Strengthening Exercises

1. Sitting Abduction (Level I)

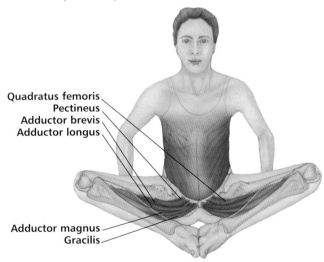

Quadratus femoris
Pectineus
Adductor brevis
Adductor longus

Adductor magnus
Gracilis

Figure 8.14: Sitting abduction.

TECHNIQUE

Sitting with a straight back, place hands on outside of thighs. Press thighs out while hands press in. Hold for 10 counts, then repeat. The abductors are on the back side of the thighs and working against resistance of the hands, while the adductors are stretching.

The Anatomy of Exercise & Movement

2. *Pilates Side Circles With Rotation* (Level I)

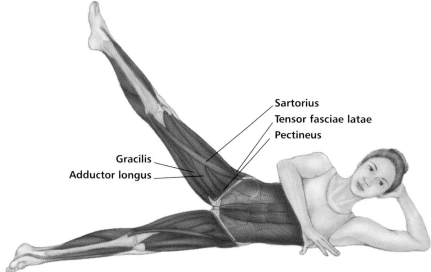

Figure 8.15: Pilates side circles with rotation.

TECHNIQUE

Lie on one side, rest head on arm or hand, with other hand on floor in front of chest. The head and neck need to be in line with spine in 'hand held' position, and the core engaged. Lift top leg, keeping the knee straight and forward. Hold, extending leg long; do not lift any higher than halfway (45 degrees). From above position, rotate leg out (knee facing up) then in (knee facing down). Repeat 5–8 times, then change sides. The Pilates **side circles** (above position completing five small circles of the leg in each direction) are also ideal for the abductors and outward rotators.

3. *Weighted Leg Lifts* (Levels I–II)

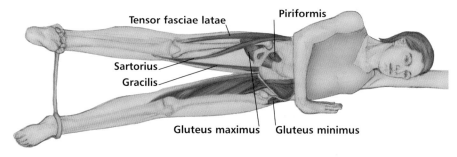

Figure 8.16: Weighted leg lifts (levels I–II).

TECHNIQUE

Assume position of side leg lifts (#2) adding ankle weights of 2–5 lbs. Lower and lift the top leg, repeating until muscle is fatigued. The leg can be parallel or turned out or in.

Alternatively, this can be done standing, holding on to a ballet barre or chair for support, lifting leg out to the side, keeping knee forward so that the leg is parallel. Cables can also be used by fastening the cuff to the ankle and lifting the leg out to the side against the resistance.

4. *Side Leg Press* (Level I)

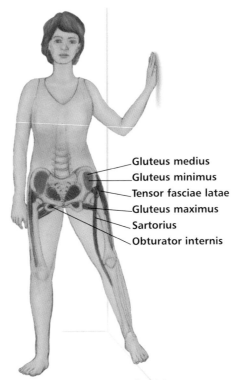

Figure 8.17: Side leg press (level I).

TECHNIQUE

Stand next to a wall 2 feet away, with left side facing wall, left hand on the wall. Lift left leg out to side until foot touches wall. Press outside of foot against the wall, keeping knee straight, and hold for at least 10 counts. Repeat on the other side. This will strengthen the abductors on both legs; the supporting leg is working just as hard, both in isometric contraction.

5. *Leg Abduction* (Level III)

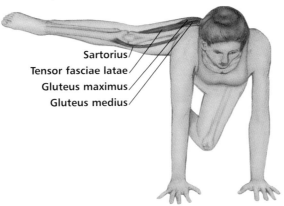

Figure 8.18: Leg abduction (level III).

TECHNIQUE

Kneeling with hands or elbows on floor directly under shoulders (all-fours), raise one leg out to the side with knee bent, until it is parallel to the floor. To increase difficulty, straighten the leg while trying to retain the same height of the thigh. Hold for 10 counts. Center body weight on both arms and do not allow leg to move forward – the hip and knee should be in a straight line.

The Anatomy of Exercise & Movement

Range of motion is limited when the leg is abducted. This is because bone hits bone: the head of the femur hits the edge of the acetabulum of the pelvis, and keeps the leg from going higher. This is bypassed when the leg rotates outward, which allows the femur to turn in the socket for increased range of motion. This is one reason why ballet is based on outward rotation of the hip: to allow the leg to lift higher. When it does, the strong hip flexors help hold the leg as the hip moves closer to flexion (thigh anterior of the pelvis) and it rotates. To isolate the abductors, the leg must be kept neutral, not rotated.

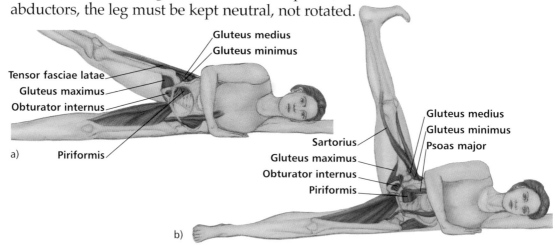

Figure 8.19: a) Abduction, b) outward rotation.

Abductors work when standing, to keep the legs stabilized underneath. While doing squats this is also happening, with added resistance of gravity, weights, or both. When standing on one foot or walking, they stabilize the pelvis. The abductors work in many standing Yoga positions, such as **vrksasana (tree pose)**.

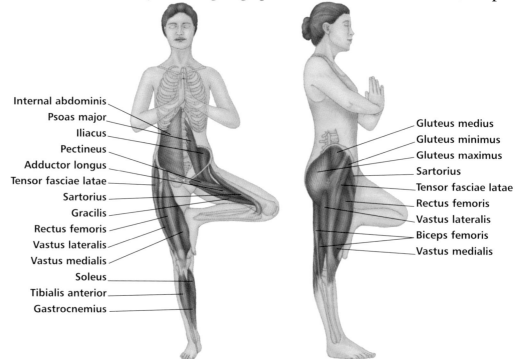

Figure 8.20: Vrksasana (tree pose).

Hip Abductor Stretching Exercises

Since the main action of these three muscles is abduction, then to stretch the muscle one must do the opposite action, which is adduction, bringing the leg toward or across the midline of the body. Any exercise that lengthens the outside of the thigh where the abductors are located will accomplish an abductor stretch.

1. *Supine Thigh Cross* (Level I)

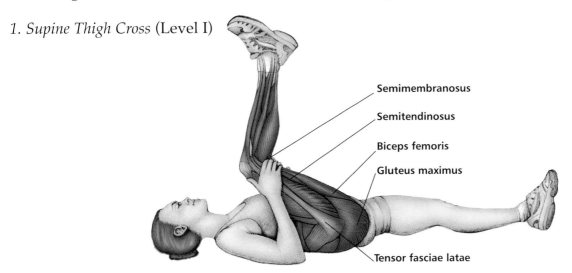

Figure 8.21: Supine thigh cross (level I).

TECHNIQUE

Lie on back with right knee into chest, left leg bent or extended on floor. Pull right knee toward left shoulder with right hand. Keep both hips on the floor. The thigh crosses the chest.

2. *Diagonal Leg Cross* (Level II)

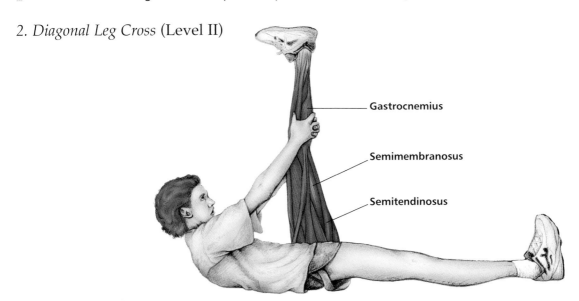

Figure 8.22: Diagonal leg cross (level II).

TECHNIQUE

Assume position in Exercise #1 and straighten the leg. The head can also be down and resting, while the left leg is stretched diagonally across to the opposite shoulder.

The Anatomy of Exercise & Movement

3. Straight Leg Cross (Level II–III)

TECHNIQUE

Assume position in Exercise #2 and take leg to the floor toward the opposite hand, arms out to sides.

The above three exercises can be done in sequence before switching to the other side.

A **combined stretch for all three glutei**, as well as most other hip joint muscles, is one that does not seem to have a name. Sometimes it is referred to as the **piriformis stretch** (the piriformis is a small, deep hip rotator described on page 152).

4. Piriformis or Crossed Leg Stretch (Level II)

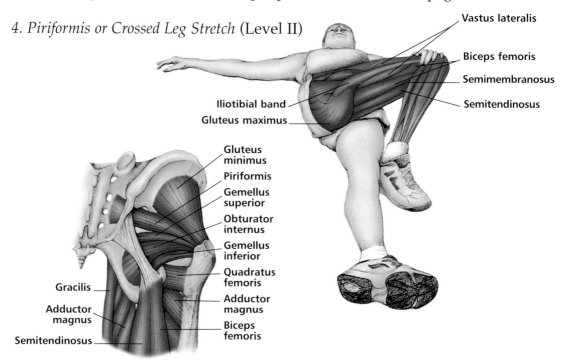

Figure 8.23: Crossed leg stretch (level II). Inset, right leg, posterior view.

TECHNIQUE

Lie on back, crossing one leg over the other knee to knee, with bottom foot still on the floor, arms out to side. Roll legs slowly to one side, then to the other. Continue the slow-motion rock as the legs get closer to the floor, then hold to one side and breathe. Switch legs and repeat. The bottom leg should be bent with foot on floor to enhance the stretch as the legs are rolled to the side.

5. Karate Kicks (Level III)

Do not be surprised that this would be considered a Level III exercise; most people would have trouble balancing on one leg while forcefully kicking out with the other and not being able to hold on to anything.

The strengthening and stretching exercises listed are by no means a complete list, but doing them consistently will help with any imbalances in the body.

Posterior Hip (Extensor) Muscles

Primary movers of extension: **gluteus maximus, biceps femoris, semitendinosus, semimembranosus.**

The **gluteus maximus** is the muscle most commonly referred to as the 'butt' (short for buttocks). 'Gluteus' is derived from the Greek word *gloutos*, meaning 'rump'. Contrary to popular belief, this is not the largest muscle in the human body.

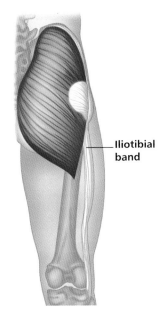

Iliotibial band

Figure 8.24: Gluteus maximus.

Working the Gluteus Maximus

The gluteus maximus is a large muscle superficial to the other two glutei, therefore seen the most. It is powerful in hip extension, which is the action that brings the thigh posterior, or behind the pelvis. Extension is also the 'return from flexion', so if the thigh is in front of the body (flexion) and returns to neutral, that is hip extension. Go from sitting (hip flexion) to standing, and hip extension has happened, with the gluteus maximus as the strongest working muscle in concentric contraction. It is eccentrically contracting going from standing to sitting,

Cardiovascular exercise such as walking, running, swimming, biking, skiing, and skating will all work the maximus. Since these exercises are aerobic, they burn body fat off naturally (pills and surgery are not natural). The magic exercise formula is 3–4 times per week, for at least 20 minutes each time: enough to reach the training heart rate and keep it at a consistent level for that amount of time. (See aerobics articles or machines to figure training rate.) Strengthening and toning the area will also happen.

A list of activities that incorporate hip extension and work the gluteus maximus are:

1. **Climbing stairs** – each time the lead foot steps and pushes 'down' to climb, the hip extends.

2. **Walking/running** – hip extension happens when the front foot pushes to propel the body forward.

3. **Jumping** – the body goes from a semi-sitting, or squat position, into the air with straight legs; the lower posterior fibers have been called "goosers".

4. **Swimming** – the breast stroke kick – a great hip extensor exercise as the legs extend to propel forward – the gluteus maximus works doubly, since the legs can be outward rotated also (a second action of the maximus).

5. **Biking** – As the leg extends, so does the hip joint.

6. **Squats** – these do the action of sitting to standing, so the maximus works hard, depending on the amount of weight used. The heavier the weight, the more work for the muscle. Some weight lifters have worked the maximus to oversized-proportions because of huge weights lifted, and then wonder how their hips got so big. Lower backs and knees can also be compromised due to too much weight and/or poor posture.

7. **Grande pliés** in dance technique classes – the gluteus maximus works in both hip extension and outward rotation on the way up from a 'squatted', turned-out position, with gravity as the resistance.

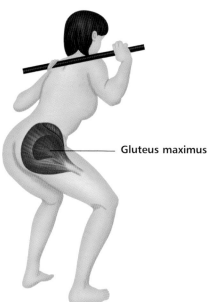

Gluteus maximus

Figure 8.25: Squats, illustrating the gluteus maximus, necessary for powerful extension of the hip.

Gluteus Maximus Strengthening Exercises

1. Setu Bandha (Bridge Pose) (Level I)
Also described as a hip flexor stretch (see page 129).

2. Posterior Leg Lifts (Level II)

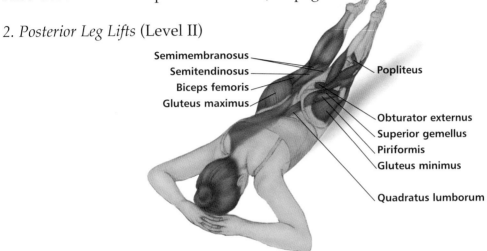

Semimembranosus
Semitendinosus
Biceps femoris
Gluteus maximus

Popliteus

Obturator externus
Superior gemellus
Piriformis
Gluteus minimus

Quadratus lumborum

Figure 8.26: Posterior leg lifts (level II).

TECHNIQUE

Lie prone and lift both legs at the same time. Keep legs hip-width apart, and the abdominals lifted against spine to support the lower back. Breathe through the ribs. Hold the position, or lift and lower. Lift one leg at a time for a Level I exercise.

Machines for the Gluteus Maximus
1. Leg Presses (Levels I–III), depending on weights used.

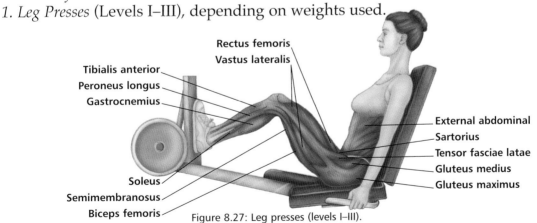

Rectus femoris
Vastus lateralis

Tibialis anterior
Peroneus longus
Gastrocnemius

External abdominal
Sartorius
Tensor fasciae latae
Gluteus medius
Gluteus maximus

Soleus
Semimembranosus
Biceps femoris

Figure 8.27: Leg presses (levels I–III).

TECHNIQUE

Keep legs parallel, or rotate outward for added benefit to the gluteus maximus.

2. Rowing Machines (Levels I–III), the longer the workout, the more beneficial the exercise, aiding the cardiovascular system as well.

3. Cable Kick Backs (Levels I–III). Level depends on weights used, and range of motion.

The Iliofemoral ("Y") Ligament

The iliofemoral ("Y") ligament in front of the hip joint limits extension and outward rotation of the hip – do not go beyond the limits imposed by this ligament! Once it is overstretched, it cannot go back to its original length, making the joint unstable. If this has already happened, extra strengthening exercises are needed to balance the joint.

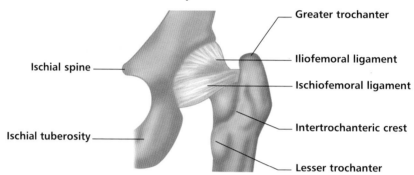

Figure 8.28: The iliofemoral ("Y") ligament.

Athletes in training have to be careful of overdoing certain movements. A ballet dancer does many plies every day just to warm up, and then jumps. Figure skaters can jump at least fifty times in a single lesson. Many weight lifters overdo the weight amount in squats. Basketball players run and jump for hours. Depending on training, hips can get 'too large', or disproportionate to the rest of the body. **Stretching afterward may help to lengthen instead of 'bulk' the muscle.**

Gluteus Maximus Stretching Exercises

1. Child's Pose (Level I)
See figure 5.13.

2. Supine Spinal Twists (Levels I–III)

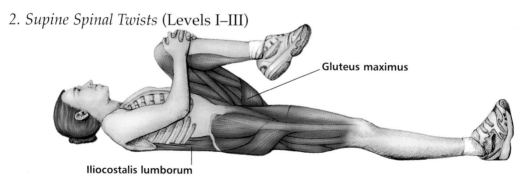

Figure 8.29: Supine spinal twists (levels I–III).

TECHNIQUE

Lie on back with legs extended. Pull left knee into chest, then allow knee to stretch toward the right shoulder (use right hand to help pull). Release left leg all the way to the right by rotating the spine, arms out to the sides. Breathe deeply, relaxing into the stretch. Repeat on the other side. Straightening the left leg is Level III.

3. Uttanasana (Standing Forward Bend) (Levels II–III)

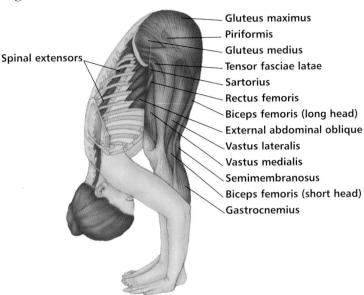

Figure 8.30: Uttanasana (standing forward bend).

TECHNIQUE

Standing with feet hip-width apart, roll head and trunk down toward the floor. Keep knees soft with weight forward toward the balls of the feet. Allow arms and head to extend in line with the torso, breathing deeply. Roll back up slowly through each vertebra, using abdominals against spine. Do not 'lock' the knees. The stomach and thighs connect to stimulate the organs, while the body elongates passively. If this sounds impossible, try bending the knees more.

4. Paschimottanasana (Seated Forward Bend) (Level III)

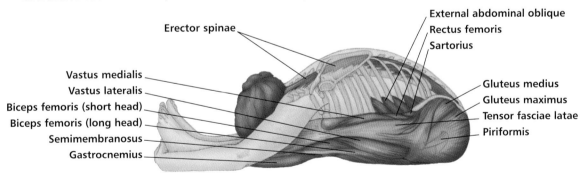

Figure 8.31: Paschimottanasana (seated forward bend).

TECHNIQUE

Sit with legs stretched straight out in front, with hands reaching toward toes. If the knees are bent it affects the gluteus maximus more than the hamstrings. The spine is extended. The seated forward bend is also a good stretch for the back extensor muscles, and when the knees are straight, the hamstrings.

The Anatomy of Exercise & Movement

The **hamstring** muscle group is also powerful in hip extension, with the three muscles forming the shape of the back of the thigh.

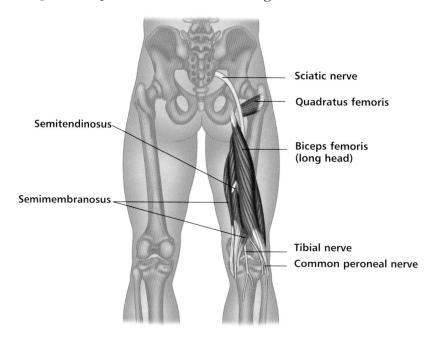

Figure 8.32: The hamstring muscle group; biceps femoris, semitendinosus and semimembranosus.

The **biceps femoris** is the most lateral of the three hamstring muscles, and usually the largest. It has two heads (the meaning of 'biceps'), the long and short heads. It is the long head that crosses the hip joint to work it. It can also contract to help in hip outward rotation.

The other two hamstrings, **semitendinosus** and **semimembranosus**, are completely synergistic, meaning they both do the exact same actions, so they can be discussed together. Working at the hip, they extend and are active in internal rotation, the opposite rotational action of the biceps femoris. Although all three hamstring muscles proximally attach at the same point on the pelvis, the ischial tuberosities, they split at the knee. The biceps femoris attaches below the outside of the knee (fibula), and the two semis attach on the inside below the knee (tibia).

All three hamstring muscles are biarticulate, or **polyarticular**, working two joints: the hip and knee. Their main action at the knee is flexion, or bending the knee.

Hip Extensor Strengthening Exercises

Hip extensor strengthening and stretching exercises discussed under the gluteus maximus section can be done for the hamstrings also. Squats and grande pliés tend to isolate and work the gluteus maximus more, while hamstrings work more in walking than the gluteus maximus does. The hamstrings can be isolated from the gluteus maximus by doing the following:

1. Lying Leg Curls (Levels I–III), depending on weights

TECHNIQUE

Lie on stomach (prone) and bend one knee at a time, adding ankle weights for more resistance. This can also be done on leg curl machines, designed in standing, sitting, or prone positions. When done on the floor, once the knee is bent, the thigh can be lifted off the floor, activating the gluteus maximus.

2. Pilates Single Leg Kicks (Levels I–II)

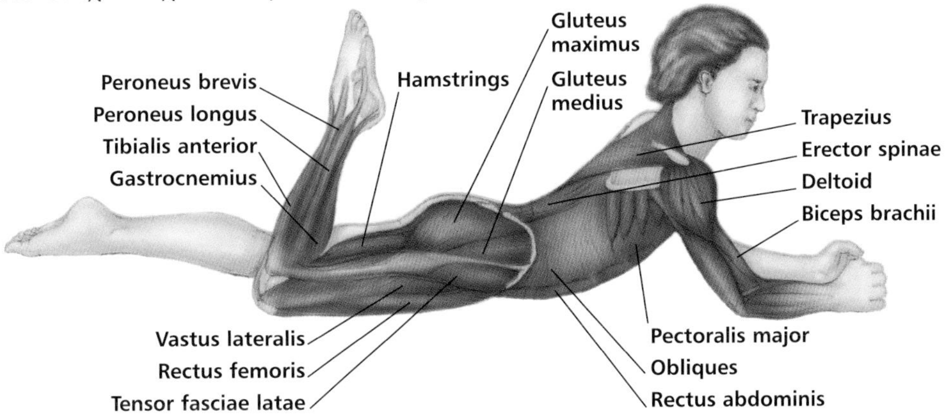

Figure 8.33: Pilates single leg kicks (levels I–II).

TECHNIQUE

Lie on stomach and lift chest with forearms on floor, elbows bent under shoulders and hands fisted. Support the lower back by lifting the abdominals, not hips, off the floor. Bend one leg with foot flexed, then switch. Repeat several times.

3. Good Mornings (Levels I–III), depending on bar weight (see figure 3.18)

TECHNIQUE

Stand with feet hip-width apart and bend trunk forward, keeping the spine straight. Return to standing position. Knees straight (not hyperextended) will isolate the hamstrings; knees bent will work the gluteus maximus. This exercise also works the spine extensors (see Chapter 3). Because all three hamstrings attach to the ischial tuberosities (sit bones), they can pull the rear pelvis down. This happens in **good mornings** with knees straight.

To separate the hip extensors from each other in fitness centers or at home on cardiovascular machines, use treadmills for the hamstrings (forward motion) and stair-climbing or elliptical for the gluteus maximus (up and down motions).

Adding outward rotation of the hip to any extensor exercise will work the gluteus maximus and biceps femoris. Doing inward rotation of the hip will isolate the semitendinosus and the semimembranosus. Hip rotation is discussed at the end of this chapter.

The Anatomy of Exercise & Movement

Hip Extensor Stretching Exercises

Stretches that incorporate a straight knee with the leg in front of the body will elongate the hamstrings fully. When the knees soften, or bend, the hamstrings are released from their line of pull at the knee and the gluteus maximus will stretch more.

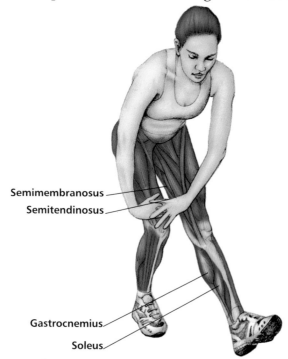

Semimembranosus
Semitendinosus

Gastrocnemius
Soleus

Figure 8.34: Standing toe-raised hamstring stretch.

TECHNIQUE

Stand with one knee bent and the other leg straight out in front. Point toes toward body and lean forward. Keep back straight and rest hands on bent knee.

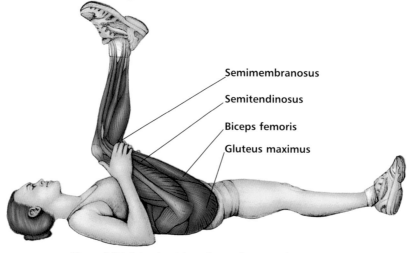

Semimembranosus

Semitendinosus

Biceps femoris

Gluteus maximus

Figure 8.35: Lying bent knee hamstring stretch.

TECHNIQUE

Lie on the back (supine) and bend one leg. Pull the other knee toward chest, then slowly and gently straighten raised leg.

In the previous exercises the hamstrings are fully engaged in the stretch because the knees are straight. Stretches to isolate the other hip extensor, the gluteus maximus, are found under that section (see pages 142/143 for gluteus maximus stretches).

Medial Hip (Adductor) Muscles

Primary movers of adduction: **pectineus, adductor magnus, adductor brevis, adductor longus, gracilis.**

These muscles shape the inside of the thigh. The adductors are similar to 'five fingers' with the 'thumb' at the top of the inside thigh, and the 'pinky' at the bottom. As the femur drops down from the lateral side of the pelvis it angles inward to the knee. This creates a 'space' inside the upper thigh that the adductor muscles fill.

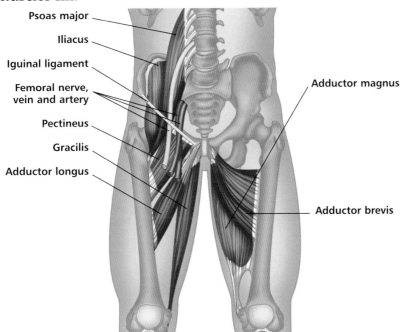

Psoas major

Iliacus

Iguinal ligament

Femoral nerve, vein and artery

Pectineus

Gracilis

Adductor longus

Adductor magnus

Adductor brevis

Figure 8.36: Medial hip (adductor) muscles.

The **pectineus** is the most superior adductor, referred to as the 'groin' area. It has already been identified as a secondary mover of hip flexion. Its primary action is adduction, or bringing the thigh toward the midline of the body.

The three muscles specifically named **adductors** are the **adductor magnus, brevis** and **longus**. They travel down the inside of the thigh, starting at the anterior pubis area of the pelvis and attaching to the medial length of the femur. The magnus is the largest of the three, as the name implies, and spreads out to cover the fullest area of the inside thigh. It has an anterior and posterior section – the space between the two distal attachments is called the adductor hiatus.

The long and slender **gracilis** attaches from the pubis symphysis to the tibia below the knee. It shapes the superficial inner thigh, but is relatively weak. It is the only biarticulate adductor muscle, working the knee as well as the hip. Most adductors also rotate the hip. The pectineus and gracilis inwardly rotate, and the adductor brevis and magnus outwardly rotate. All adductors function as stabilizers of the leg when weight is on it; they help keep the legs underneath the body. They also stabilize the pelvis.

Hip Adductor Strengthening Exercises

1. *Bottom Leg Lifts* (Levels I–II)

Bottom leg lifts are the most popular adductor exercise, done in Pilates and many floor exercise classes.

TECHNIQUE

Lie on one side with head resting on bottom arm, top hand on the floor in front of chest or holding onto the ankle. The top leg is bent in front so the bottom leg is free to move. Lift and lower bottom leg 5–8 times; add ankle weights, rotation, or leg circles for a harder workout. Always repeat on the other side.

2. *Sitting Adduction* (Level 1)

TECHNIQUE

Sit straight in a chair with legs hip-width apart. Place hands inside the legs and push thighs in. Added benefit: using the hands will exercise the shoulder and arm muscles while you push against the thighs.

3. *Pool Exercises* (Level I)

Exercising in a pool has the advantage of water resistance without too much impact on the body.

TECHNIQUE

a) Stand holding on to the side of the pool and cross one leg in front, then behind the body. Keep the leg outward rotated for a few repetitions, then inward rotate. Repeat on the other leg.

b) To work both legs at the same time, hold onto a diving board or the side of the pool with the spine against it. Straddle, then close the legs, repeating 8–10 times. Good for both adduction and abduction.

4. *Cable Adduction* (Level II)

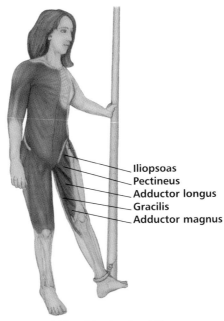

Figure 8.37: Cable adduction (level II).

TECHNIQUE

A strap is placed around the foot. The spring provides the tension as the leg crosses past the midline of the body.

With the added resistance of the spring cable attached to the foot or ankle, grasp the machine and pull the leg toward the midline, then across the other leg.

5. *Machine Adduction* (Levels II–III)

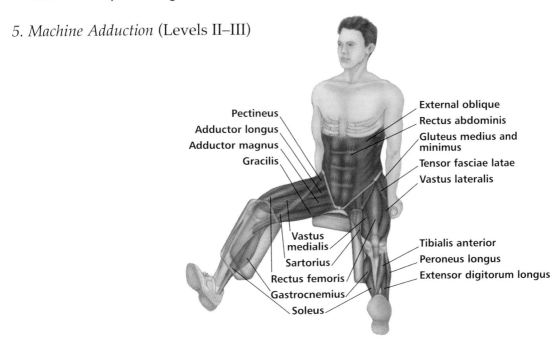

Figure 8.38: Hip adduction machine.

TECHNIQUE

Assume a sitting posture with legs wide. Resistance is applied on the inside of the thighs, as the legs push in against it. Can be held, or repeated in sets.

The Anatomy of Exercise & Movement

Hip Adductor Stretching Exercises

Any body position that puts the leg in an abducted position will stretch the adductors.

1. Baddha Konasana (Butterfly Pose) (Level I)

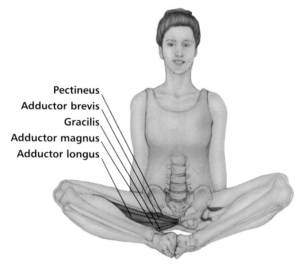

Pectineus
Adductor brevis
Gracilis
Adductor magnus
Adductor longus

Figure 8.39: Baddha konasana (butterfly pose) (level I).

TECHNIQUE

Sit and open thighs outward, with soles of feet touching each other. Hands can support the spine by being placed on floor behind hips. For added stretch, place hands on inside of knees and press down gently; rounding the spine with head toward the feet will also increase the stretch.

2. Sitting Wide Leg Stretch (Level II–III)

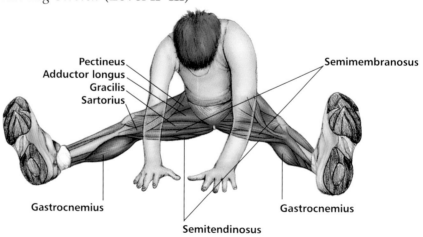

Pectineus
Adductor longus
Gracilis
Sartorius

Semimembranosus

Gastrocnemius

Gastrocnemius

Semitendinosus

Figure 8.40: Sitting wide leg stretch (level II-III).

TECHNIQUE

Sit with the legs straight and wide apart. Keep the back straight and lean forward. For level III, move the legs further apart.

3. *Upside-down Butterfly* (Levels I–II)

TECHNIQUE

Lie on back with knees into chest. Open thighs outward, soles of feet touching. Reach arms through legs and hold ankles. Pull them toward chest for added stretch, as elbows press the knees away from each other. Straighten one leg at a time out to the side for more stretch.

4. *Standing Leg-up Stretch* (Levels I–II)

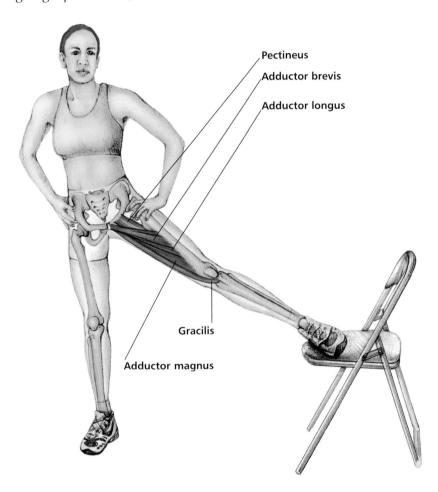

Pectineus

Adductor brevis

Adductor longus

Gracilis

Adductor magnus

Figure 8.41: Standing leg-up stretch (level I).

TECHNIQUE

Stand upright and place one leg out to the side and the foot up on a raised object. Keep the toes facing forward and slowly move the other leg away from the object. For level II, use a higher object and if you need to, hold on to something for balance.

Six Deep Rotators

Piriformis, gemellus superior and inferior, obturator internus and externus, quadratus femoris.

Located under the gluteal muscles, the six deep rotators are the smallest muscles of the hip and are primarily responsible for outward rotation. In ballet, the outward rotation of the legs so sought after has to do mostly with these little deep posterior muscles under the butt. Other larger hip muscles will help.

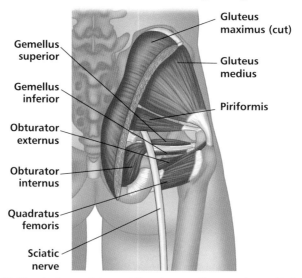

Figure 8.42: The six deep rotators; piriformis, gemellus superior and inferior, obturator internus and externus, quadratus femoris.

The **piriformis** is superior and the only one of the six attached to the sacrum, passing through the greater sciatic notch, and inserting into the greater trochanter of the femur. It outwardly rotates when the sacrum is fixed; it is also active when the pelvis 'shifts'. The path of the muscle indicates that when tight or spasmodic, it could hinder the sciatic nerve, causing what doctors term **sciatica**. This condition causes pain along the path of the nerve into the thigh, and is usually attributed to disc trouble in the lumbar area of the spine. Better to release a tight hip muscle before thinking there is a bulging disc problem.

The **gemellus superior and inferior** (the gemelli) are small, thin muscles that cross the hip joint from the area of the ischium to the greater trochanter of the femur. Their path is almost horizontal across the joint.

Lying between the two gemelli, the **obturator internus** has a broad origin on a part of the pelvis called the obturator foramen, along with portions of the lower iliac bone. Fibers then pass through the lesser sciatic notch and on to the femur. Besides being an outward rotator, it is a strong stabilizer of the hip.

The **obturator externus** is an ideal rotator of the hip due to its position. It passes from the lower end of the obturator foramen, then behind the neck of the femur to attach to the greater trochanter of the femur on the medial side. Its line of pull allows the head of the femur to roll laterally inside the socket of the pelvis, creating outward, or external rotation.

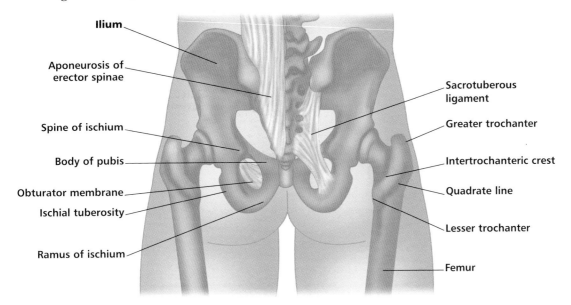

Ilium

Aponeurosis of erector spinae

Spine of ischium

Body of pubis

Obturator membrane

Ischial tuberosity

Ramus of ischium

Sacrotuberous ligament

Greater trochanter

Intertrochanteric crest

Quadrate line

Lesser trochanter

Femur

8.43: Bones of the pelvic girdle (posterior view).

The most inferior (lowest) deep rotator is the **quadratus femoris**. "Quadratus" means "square"; it is a short muscle running almost horizontal from the upper portion of the ischial tuberosity to the femur. Do not confuse this muscle with the quadriceps femoris muscle group, the extensors of the knee.

The six deep rotator muscles can pull the pelvis forward, and help balance the pelvis and spine along with the psoas. They also have minor secondary actions at the hip. The top three can extend and abduct, the bottom three can extend and adduct.

The sartorius, gluteus maximus, biceps femoris, and three adductors also help the six deep rotators in outward rotation. With so many muscles capable of one action, strengthening and stretching is very important. (It is easiest to isolate the rotators by freeing the leg from support on the floor.)

Outward Rotator Strengthening Exercises

1. *Sitting/Lying Leg Rotation* (Level I)

TECHNIQUE

Sitting straight in a chair with hands on the sides, extend both legs out in front, heels together. Rotate legs out, then in. Very easy, and a good way to find and feel the muscles working. Try to lift the torso so the weight is 'up' in the chair, and 'squeeze the butt together'. This activates small pelvic floor muscles. This can also be done sitting on the floor, or in supine position with the legs toward the ceiling.

2. *Standing Leg Rotation* (Level I)

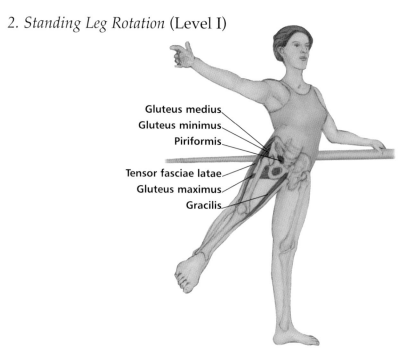

Gluteus medius
Gluteus minimus
Piriformis
Tensor fasciae latae
Gluteus maximus
Gracilis

Figure 8.44: Standing leg rotation (level I). (Shows internal rotation.)

TECHNIQUE

Holding on to the wall or barre with one hand, lift outside leg to the side a few inches off the floor, keeping the hip down. Rotate out and in. Try it higher, but not above 45 degrees.

3. *Rond de Jambe* (Levels I–III)

TECHNIQUE

A ballet exercise executed standing; this is done by extending one leg forward, side, then back in a continuous circular movement, maintaining outward rotation throughout. Toes on the floor is level I, off the floor is level II. Harder than it seems, try lifting the leg to waist height (level III). Ballet is not easy!

Outward Rotator Stretching Exercises

One must inward rotate to stretch the outward rotators. When the legs are crossed, the bottom leg is slightly inward rotated. Try the **crossed leg stretch** (see page 138) with the lower leg bent. It is one of the best stretches for the top of the six deep rotators, the piriformis. Remember, this muscle is a culprit in 'sciatica', a term used when the sciatic nerve is restricted. A tight piriformis will affect the nerve, causing discomfort and/or pain in the hip and thigh. The ability to relax and elongate this muscle is simple; think of the medical bills one can save. Also try the **sitting foot-to-chest buttocks stretch**.

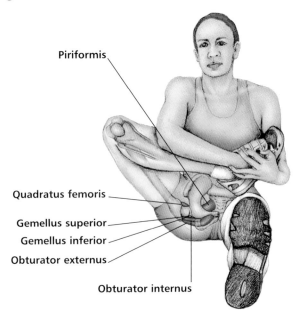

Piriformis

Quadratus femoris

Gemellus superior

Gemellus inferior

Obturator externus

Obturator internus

Figure 8.45: Sitting foot-to-chest buttocks stretch.

TECHNIQUE

Sit with one leg straight and hold onto the other ankle, pulling it directly toward the chest. Use the hands and arms to regulate the intensity of the stretch. The closer you pull the foot to the chest, the more intense the stretch.

Inward Rotators of the Hip

Don't panic, these muscles have already been covered. They are: **gluteus medius and minimus, tensor fasciae latae, semitendinosus, semimembranosus, gracilis, pectineus** (according to most sources).

Most exercises for outward (external) rotation can be reversed to inward (internal) rotation; just roll the thigh in instead of out.

Hip Imbalances

Everyone has them. Scenarios:

1) One hip might be tighter than the other simply because of standing on one leg more.

2) Physical activity that demands strength of the lower extremity, such as running and cycling, needs more stretching to alleviate tight muscles.

3) Any sport where the ideal is a flexible, high leg (dance, figure skating, rhythmic gymnastics) might lead to an unstable joint unless strength exercises are done to counteract the looseness.

There are no 'double joints', just very loose ones. The hip area may be extensive, but it houses the central basin of the body and connects to the legs. Respect it.

Myths of the Iliofemoral (Hip) Joint Dispelled

Most muscles of the hip do more than one action at the hip
This is true of all ball-and-socket joints, and the hip is no exception. Of all the large muscles around the iliofemoral joint, the rectus femoris is the only muscle that can do only one action at the hip: flexion. Of course, it is also a quadriceps muscle, therefore can extend the knee as well. The fourteen other large muscles can each do other actions. The six deep rotators externally rotate, but these are small muscles and do have some secondary work. **It is easy to confuse the rectus femoris and quadratus femoris because of the names. The rectus is a large, anterior, biarticulate muscle; the quadratus femoris is one of the six small, deep rotators found posteriorly, inferior to the other five. They both work the hip joint differently.**

Hip imbalance can be corrected
There is some great postural work that can aid anyone to help keep the hip in balance. Most hip replacements happen because bone has worn away bone. Pressure can be kept off the shock absorbers between the bones (cartilage) if the femur and pelvis are properly aligned, and the weight of the body is distributed well. Too much weight will hinder the effectiveness of the joint. **Patients with (or without!) joint surgery need to maintain a good weight for their bone structure; doctors can help to enforce this.**

The weekend athlete
Be wary of becoming a 'weekend athlete'; stay conditioned throughout the week to keep from shocking the body and specifically, the joints. Also, one must be careful of overuse for too many years. **Lifetime sports can be great if care is taken to keep from getting injured repeatedly. In summary, hip replacement can be avoided!**

Main Muscles Involved in Movements of the Iliofemoral (Hip) Joint

Flexion
Iliopsoas; Rectus Femoris; Tensor Fasciae Latae; Sartorius; Adductor Brevis; Adductor Longus; Pectineus

Extension
Gluteus Maximus; Semitendinosus; Semimembranosus; Biceps Femoris (long head); Adductor Magnus (ischial fibers)

Abduction
Gluteus Medius; Gluteus Minimus; Tensor Fasciae Latae; Obturator Internus (in flexion); Piriformis (in flexion)

Adduction
Adductor Magnus; Adductor Brevis; Adductor Longus; Pectineus; Gracilis; Gluteus Maximus (lower fibers); Quadratus Femoris

Lateral Rotation
Gluteus Maximus; Obturator Internus; Gemelli; Obturator Externus; Quadratus Femoris; Piriformis; Sartorius; Adductor Magnus; Adductor Brevis; Adductor Longus; Biceps Femoris

Medial Rotation
Tensor Fasciae Latae; Gluteus Medius (anterior fibers); Gluteus Minimus (anterior fibers); Semitendinosus; Semimembranosus; Gracilis

The Knee Joint

Knees are a perfect example of a joint: two bones articulated (joined), held together by ligaments, with muscle tendons attached to move the joint, cartilage to absorb shock, and synovial fluid inside a membrane to lubricate. It is the largest joint in the body, with the two long bones (femur and tibia) acting as levers; where they meet there is little lateral movement.

The Anatomy of Exercise & Movement

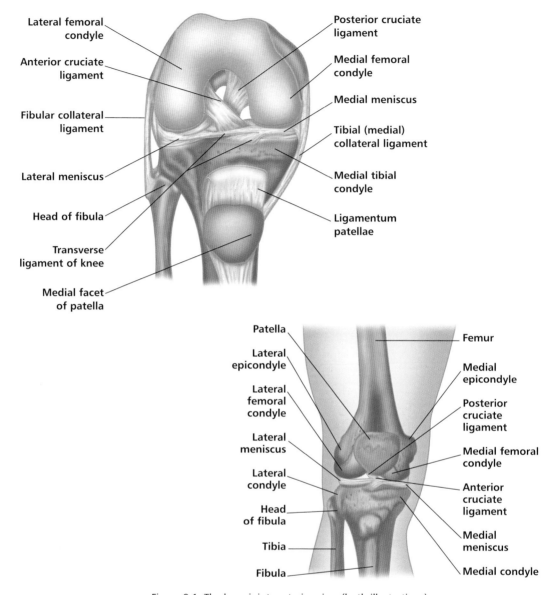

Figure 9.1: The knee joint, anterior view (both illustrations).

The two collateral ligaments are shown on the sides of the knee, known as the tibial (medial) collateral and fibular (lateral) collateral ligaments. The anterior and posterior cruciate ligaments cross each other inside the knee joint. Cartilage (medial and lateral meniscus) is pictured between the two bones, the femur and the tibia. The patella (knee cap) has been removed in the illustration to view the deeper parts.

The knee joint contains several bursae, sacs filled with a viscid fluid, which reduce friction by acting as a cushion for the joint. The deep bursa formed by the joint capsule at the knee, the suprapatellar bursa, is the largest bursa in the body. It is located between the femur and quadriceps femoris tendon. Three other major bursae of the knee are the subcutaneous prepatellar bursa, located between the skin and the anterior surface of the patella, the superficial infrapatellar bursa, located between the skin and the patellar tendon, and the deep infrapatellar bursa, located between the tibial tuberosity and the patellar tendon. Finally, the pes anserinus bursa is located at the lower inside of the knee joint, where sartorius, gracilis, and semitendinosus insert as the conjoined pes anserinus tendon.

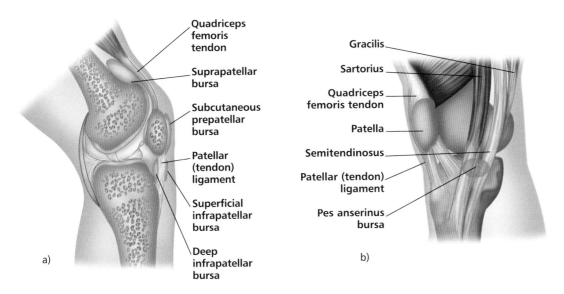

Figure 9.2: The knee joint; a) mid-sagittal view, b) medial view.

Add the patella and its ligament that extends from the quadriceps tendon, the fibula as an anchor for tendons and ligaments, and two rotary actions to mobilize the joint, and it becomes more complicated. The knee is a highly specialized mechanism of design. Imagine the knee joint without the patella to protect it anteriorly, or the cruciate and collateral ligaments to stabilize it. Some people have abused their knees so much that they are actually walking around without the aid of all this built-in protection. Ligaments and cartilage are stretched, torn, or worn; muscles are weak; bones are out of alignment. Long-term dysfunction is tolerated until pain becomes unbearable.

Hence the marvel of modern medicine: knee replacement! A miraculous surgery for some, but for others it can be avoided. With correct therapy, strength and postural work, the pain can be eased and the body balanced without the invasion of surgery.

If conditions are dealt with early on, joint replacement can be avoided.

Knee Extensors: Quadriceps Femoris

The famous "quads" are a group of four muscles that work together to do one main movement: extension (straightening) of the knee. *The four quadriceps muscles are:* **rectus femoris, vastus medialis, vastus intermedius, vastus lateralis.**

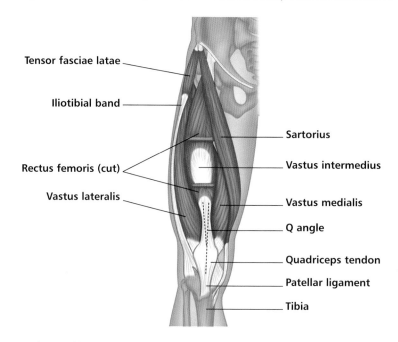

Tensor fasciae latae

Iliotibial band

Rectus femoris (cut)

Vastus lateralis

Sartorius

Vastus intermedius

Vastus medialis

Q angle

Quadriceps tendon

Patellar ligament

Tibia

Figure 9.3: The quadriceps muscles. (The Q angle is delineated, and described on the next page.)

The quadricep muscles are active in many movements: walking, running, jumping, kicking; any movement that straightens the knee. It is the most powerful and largest muscle group in the human body. The quadriceps are stronger than their antagonists, the hamstrings. It is desirable to have the quads approximately 20% stronger to balance the mechanisms of the knee joint.

They are the only extensors of the knee, but two of them also contribute to the rotational movement of the lower leg. The vastus medialis inward rotates, and the vastus lateralis outward rotates, only when the knee is flexed. No rotation is possible when the knee is straight.

The most superficial of the quadriceps, the rectus femoris, is also the only one that can work two joints (biarticulate). Described in Chapter 8 as a hip flexor, it travels down the front of the thigh to insert with the other three quad muscles into a common quadriceps tendon. This tendon passes over the patella into the tibia as the patellar ligament.

While the four quadriceps concentrically contract together to straighten the knee when jumping, they also act as brakes upon landing, eccentrically contracting while the knees bend to keep the body from collapsing to the ground. This makes them the main knee mover of the entire jump.

The Q angle is the line of pull of the quadriceps on the patella. As one can see in Figure 9.3, this is not vertical. A line drawn from the patella to the ASIS intersects with a line from the femur through the patella to the tibial tuberosity. This determines the angle, with normal ranging between 10 and 17 degrees. It is usually higher in females. Larger angles can lead to problems because of the increased off-center pull.

The shaft of the femur is also not vertical, but the center of the hip joint is almost directly in line with the center of the knee joint. This is called the mechanical axis of the femur and is crucial to proper transmission of weight through the leg.

Quadriceps Strengthening Exercises

Machines: **Leg presses, knee extensions, rowing**, any cardiovascular equipment where the knee extends against resistance, promotes concentric contraction.
Isometric contractions of a straight leg against an immoveable force (a wall or floor).
Weights: **Barbell plié squats** (illustrated below).
Ballet: **Grande pliés** and **front battements**.
Pilates: **The frog** on the reformer.

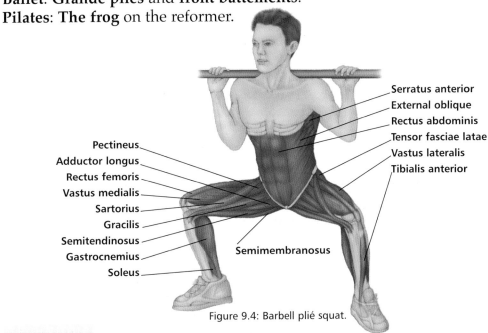

Serratus anterior
External oblique
Rectus abdominis
Tensor fasciae latae
Vastus lateralis
Tibialis anterior

Pectineus
Adductor longus
Rectus femoris
Vastus medialis
Sartorius
Gracilis
Semitendinosus
Gastrocnemius
Soleus

Semimembranosus

Figure 9.4: Barbell plié squat.

To perform correctly, avoid momentum by using slow, controlled movement. Keep the chest open, and avoid rounding the shoulders. Keep the weight directly over the heel to mid-foot, and keep the knees from passing over the vertical line of the toes. Prevent the knees and ankles from rolling inward. Squats can also be done in parallel position (feet pointed forward); repetitions and sets are usually done. The quads are maximally strengthened on the way up. Knee alignment and correct weight are important to prevent injury.

For rectus femoris:
The muscle can be isolated when the hip is flexed with a straight knee against gravity. In a sitting position with legs in out in front, bend trunk slightly forward and lift one leg a few inches off the floor for 10 seconds. The rectus muscle will feel firm; fatigue will happen shortly.

For vastus medialis:
Sit on a chair and stabilize the feet by placing a block between them on the floor. Keeping the thigh straight, rotate the lower legs in toward the block and hold the contraction for 10 seconds. Repeat until fatigue is felt.

For vastus medialis and lateralis:
Remove block and rotate lower leg in and out, keeping the thigh still. Add ankle weights for more resistance and do knee extensions for all quads. Many Yoga postures also work the quadriceps, such as **virabhadrasanas, trikonasanas, uttanasanas** (with knees straight), and **downward facing dog**.

Quadriceps Stretching Exercises

1) **Bridge pose** (also a stretch for the abdominals).
2) **Lunges** – the stretch for the knee extensors is in the back leg. If the knee is bent to the floor and the pelvis pushed forward, the stretch will increase.
3) The rectus femoris will stretch when the hip is extended and the knee is flexed, as in **bow pose** from Yoga.
4) The vasti muscles will stretch whenever the knee is flexed.

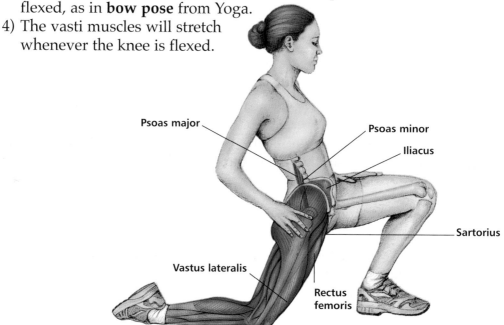

Figure 9.5: The kneeling quad stretch.
From a lunge position, rest back knee on floor. If needed, hold on to something to keep balance. Push hips forward. If need be, place a towel or mat under knee for comfort.

Knee Flexors: The Hamstrings

The flexors of the knee are commonly known as the **hamstrings**, covered in Chapter 8 as hip extensors, and therefore biarticulate. Contrary to popular belief, they are not the only knee flexors. Five other muscles aid the three hamstrings to bend the knee: the **sartorius, gracilis, popliteus, gastrocnemius,** and **plantaris** (the last two are weak knee flexors).

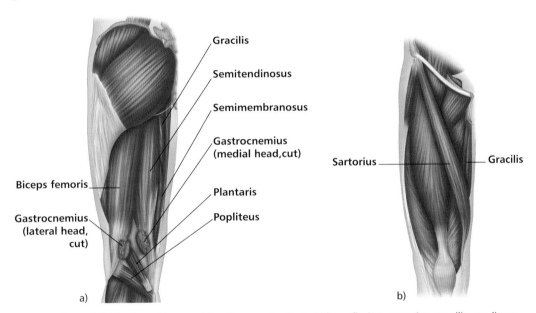

Figure 9.6: The hamstrings and the five muscles that aid knee flexion, sartorius, gracilis, popliteus, gastrocnemius, plantaris; a) posterior view, b) anterior view.

The only flexor that can outward rotate the knee is the biceps femoris of the hamstring group. Inward rotators are the semitendinosus, semimembranosus (both hamstrings), the sartorius, popliteus and gracilis. These rotational movements are vital to the knee's ability to adapt to directional changes.

Of the eight knee flexors, popliteus is the only one that is not biarticulate. Working only the knee, it is essential to the stability of the posterior aspect. It can check knee hyperextension, making it invaluable in correcting a common postural problem. Hyperextension is a straight leg that has gone past vertical, sometimes bowing the leg. One of the most important lessons in movement: don't lock the knees! In most individuals when this happens, ligaments and tendons have been over-stretched by physically bracing, or locking the knee when trying to straighten it, pushing the kneecap out of alignment. In a smaller number of cases, hyperextension is apparent from birth, usually due to bone or tissue placement.

There is a simple postural cure for hyperextended knees: when the knee is straight, do not force it beyond normal. The back of the knee should be 'soft' and not fully

The Anatomy of Exercise & Movement

stretched. The leg will look straight but will not lock past vertical. This alignment process is important; it places the weight of the leg over the correct bone in the ankle, the talus, so body weight is transferred properly through the foot.

Correct alignment of the knees between the ankle and the hip is necessary for proper function of the entire musculo-skeletal system.

Knee Flexor Strengthening Exercises

Machines: Leg curls; any cardiovascular equipment where the knee flexes against resistance, promoting concentric contraction.
Isometric contractions of a bent leg against an immoveable force.
Weights: Back leg lifts with ankle weights – if knees are bent the level increases.
Pilates: Single and double leg kicks.
Ballet: Back battements – bend the knee as in an "attitude" and all knee flexors will work.
Yoga: Bridge, camel, upward facing dog (hamstrings only), **virabhadrasana III** (bend the back leg for added strength work).

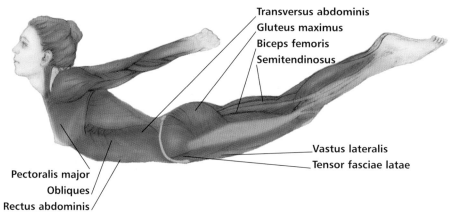

Figure 9.7: Pilates double leg kicks.

Lie on the stomach, head turned to the side, legs together, and feet pointed. Clasp the hands behind the back, placing them as high up the spine as possible. Keep the elbows wide, and touching the mat. Bend both knees and kick them toward the bottom. Stretch the clamped hands out behind you, reaching down the back, and simultaneously, raise the legs off the mat. The head and chest can be lifted off the floor for added challenge, then returned to starting position.

Knee Flexor Stretching Exercises

Stretching the hamstrings can be achieved in any exercise that lengthens them by either flexing the hip, straightening the knee, or both. Gluteus maximus stretches from Chapter 8 will stretch the hamstrings, as well as any forward bend (standing or sitting). One of the best stretches is the **lying straight knee hamstring stretch**.

Lie down on the back with one leg straight up, applying a strap or band around the foot and pulling the leg toward the chest with as straight a knee as possible.

Other flexors, such as the popliteus and gastrocnemius, can best be stretched by standing in a lunge, straightening the back knee while the heel remains on the floor.

Knee Injuries

The knee's location between the hip and the ankle make it a weight-bearing joint that is extremely vulnerable. A reminder that the human species developed from all fours to two legs; this exposed the two knee joints to constant stress. Due to many injuries, research into knee dynamics has increased and much is still being discovered. Some of the more prevalent knee conditions are described below.

ACL (Anterior Cruciate Ligament) Tears

New information on anterior cruciate ligament tears, particularly in women, has surfaced over the past few years. Research is trying to establish differences between men and women's knees as being the culprit; maybe it is just that there are finally more female athletes who need to be conditioned as well as their male counterparts have historically been. That being said, there is some validity to the anatomical argument.

1) The inlet of the female pelvic bone can be larger than a male's (for bearing children). This may make the pelvis wider, increasing the angle of the femur from the hip to the knee (the Q angle ratio discussed earlier). Research to date has not found this to be an important factor in the high percentage of ACL tears.

2) Focus is turning to the hamstrings. This muscle group aids the ACL in keeping the tibia from going forward beneath the femur, commonly called **anterior tibial translation**. There is a theory that the female quadriceps muscle group (antagonistic to the hamstrings) recruits faster than the hamstrings by a split second when the tibia is forced forward. This would place more stress on the ACL in the initial movement phase.

3) Hormonal changes can have an effect on body mechanics. During childbearing, hormones are released (relaxin) that can loosen tissue. Hormones are also influenced by the birth control pill. Studies are currently inconclusive as to the effect of hormone changes during the monthly cycle on the ACL.

One common sense solution to the problem is to increase the strength and speed of the hamstrings. If the hamstrings are less than 60% as strong as the quads, there is an imbalance and possibility of injury. After measuring knee strength in many kinesiology students over the past years, this author has found much weaker hamstrings in relation to quads (less than 60/100) in women, especially dancers. To increase strength in the hamstrings it is best to isolate them from the stronger gluteus maximus in hip extension. Leg curls are a great way to do this, but an exercise that dancers usually do not do. (Dancers need to spend more time in the weight room!)

To increase speed, there are a series of movement patterns that can be practiced, such as lunges, hopping combinations, and jumping exercises to 'retrain' the biomechanics of the leg in fast-moving combinations. **Plyometrics** is a great training tool.

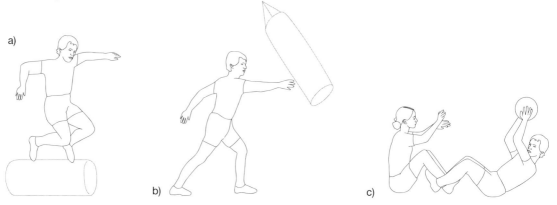

Figure 9.8: Examples of plyometric training; a) side to side jumping, b) punch bag push, c) trunk curl and throw.

Tight Hamstrings

Many people have them. Tightness can lead to imbalances in the rest of the body. Hamstrings are tight if one spends a lot of time sitting (the knees are always bent). They are also notoriously tight in athletic people who run or bike, where the hamstring muscle group works together to produce knee flexion and hip extension, therefore 'bulking' the muscle group. Tai Chi experts have tight hamstrings because the knees are in a state of constant flexion while practicing the form. Downhill skiers are also in this position throughout the length of the run.

It is an easy area to stretch: simply keep the knees as straight as possible, without locking, while bending forward (hip flexion), sitting or standing.

Stretching is a form of exercise. Exercise increases blood flow not only to the muscles, but to the brain, allowing for improved function. It is time the debate on the benefits of stretching is over.

Cartilage Wear and Tear

Cartilage wear is no longer symptomatic of only older age; it is now more prevalent than ever in younger people. The reason is the increase and impact of sports.

Two main areas of cartilage in the knee can be affected. Cartilage underneath the kneecap is ground down over a period of time by repeated use, producing **chondromalacia patellae (runner's knee).** This is most commonly found in runners and jumpers, and as much as one may enjoy manual transmission, having to constantly use a clutch while driving can cause wear under the knee. There is a grinding sensation, and as it worsens, pain and swelling.

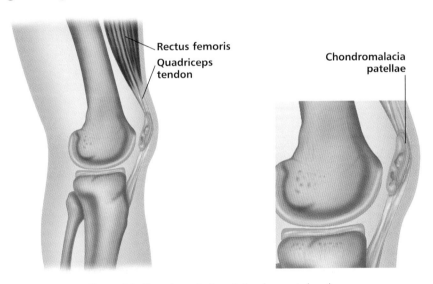

Figure 9.9: Chondromalacia patellae (runner's knee).

The placement of the patella in relation to the femur could be the cause, as well as overuse. The patella is held in place by the quadriceps tendon. If there is imbalance in strength within the four quadriceps, this could affect the placement of the kneecap. Exercising the lateral and medial vasti muscles of the quads can help align the kneecap. Through strength tests with college students, more weakness has been found in the vastus medialis than any other quadriceps muscle. This muscle not only extends but also inward rotates the knee to some extent when the knee is bent. It can be seen directly above the knee on the inside of the leg.

Meniscus Tear

The main cartilage of the knee is found between the tibia and femur and is referred to as the **meniscus**. It appears as a 'figure 8' inside the joint, with the medial meniscus thicker than the lateral. It can be worn or torn through overuse or forceful impact. Any position that involves deep knee bending can be a culprit: weight lifters doing squats, baseball catchers, goalkeepers, dancers' grande plies, track runners at the starting block, to name a few. Quick directional changes in running or skiing can also injure the meniscus. Landing on hard surfaces repeatedly, especially while wearing incorrect shoes, can deplete the effect of cartilage shock absorption.

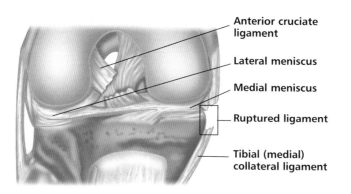
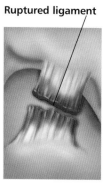

Anterior cruciate ligament

Lateral meniscus

Medial meniscus

Ruptured ligament

Tibial (medial) collateral ligament

Ruptured ligament

Ligament tear

Figure 9.10: Knee joint, anterior view. Medial (tibial) collateral ligament damage.

Articular, or hyaline cartilage protects the surface of the two bones it lies between. The large medial and smaller lateral menisci in the knee also help stabilize as well as absorb shock. When injured, a locking sensation can be felt, and if torn, extreme pain and swelling. **Keeping the knee balanced by strengthening muscles can prevent injury and surgery.**

Once cartilage is injured, limited use or complete rest can help heal the area. Some cartilage has a minute metabolism; there are tiny capillaries that supply blood to the tissue. This means it can rejuvenate itself, but the metabolism rate is extremely slow. Many people do not want to wait this long for relief. Surgery is their chosen alternative if the cartilage is torn. Less invasive surgeries are being developed that can 'clean' the inside of the knee of shredded tissue, followed by a designated exercise regimen. Clinics such as the Steadman-Hawkins Center in Vail, Colorado are doing wonderful work in the field of orthopaedics.

Collateral Ligament Damage

The most common injuries of the knee are to the ligaments. The collateral ligaments are located on the inside and outside of the knee, keeping the tibia and femur in place.

The medial, or tibial collateral ligament (MCL) takes the most abuse. Even though it is longer and larger than the lateral (fibular) collateral, it receives the most impact as blows are made against the outside of the knee, stretching the inside. This happens in contact sports where a fall results in force against the lateral side of the knee by team-mates or opponents. The medial tissue is overstretched and can even tear the inside MCL as it accepts the burden. **Stress on the ligament can affect the medial meniscus, as the deeper fibers are attached, leading to more advanced trauma.**

Ligaments do not bounce back after being overstretched. This leads to instability of the joint. **Once ligaments are unstable, the tendons of the muscles need to take over to help hold the joint together. Strength exercises for all muscles around the joint are necessary.**

Pronation of the Ankle Affects the Knee

The lower ankle joint can pronate and supinate, where weight is distributed to either side of the foot. Extreme pronation is evident when standing with the weight on the inside of the foot. This can become a chronic condition and affect the ankle, knee and hip. Ballet dancers are notorious for pronating because:

1) hip turnout has been incorrectly enforced
2) ballet shoes do not offer much support.

Besides becoming constantly aware of correct weight placement through the feet, do the following exercises:

1. **Point and flex** – Strengthen the calf muscles, especially the tibialis posterior, by pointing the foot (plantar flexion); elongate both sides of the foot through the toes. Flexing (dorsiflexion) stretches the same muscles.

2. **Calf raises** – Rise up and down on the balls of the feet with the weight placed ideally under the first three toes. Common mistake: weight is either under the little toe (supination) or the big toe only (pronation). Look in a mirror while doing the exercise to help correct alignment.

3. **Massage and exercise** the foot by rolling a tennis ball under it.

Myths of the Knee Dispelled

Only one quadricep muscle is biarticulate

The quadriceps is a group of four muscles that lie on the front of the thigh and extend the knee. The hip flexors are a group of four muscles that also lie on the front of the thigh and do flexion of the hip. The only muscle that works knee extension and hip flexion both out of these two groups is the rectus femoris. **The hip and knee share many muscles, but only one of them is a quadriceps muscle of the knee.**

The hamstrings are not the only knee flexors

The biceps femoris, semimembranosus and semitendinosus are the three individual muscles that make up the hamstring muscle group, notoriously known for flexing (bending) the knee, strongly contracting during a leg curl. There are five other knee flexors and most also work the hip or ankle joint: the sartorius and gracilis (biarticulate with the hip), and the gastrocnemius and plantaris (biarticulate with the ankle). **All knee flexors are biarticulate except for the popliteus.**

Arthritis in the knee is too common

A main cause of arthritis is too much wear and tear on a joint; this is one of the most common conditions that limit use of the knee. For years the medical profession has dealt with this problem through medications, and sometimes surgery. Twenty years ago, cartilage repair left a large zipper-like scar on the knee; and 'draining the knee' when swollen left arthritis. Although treatment techniques have advanced, the medical and pharmaceutical industries seem intent on using surgery and drugs. In some cases this is necessary, but better to condition the knee joint correctly and naturally, and achieve prevention or rehabilitation through exercise. **Arthritis is an inflammation to the joint. It has been found that low-impact aerobic activity, range of motion exercises, and strength training can ease the effects of this disease.**

Main Muscles Involved in Movements of the Knee Joint

Flexion
Semitendinosus; Semimembranosus; Biceps Femoris; Gastrocnemius; Plantaris; Sartorius; Gracilis; Popliteus

Extension
Rectus Femoris; Vastus Medialis; Vastus Lateralis; Vastus Intermedius

Medial Rotation of Tibia on Femur
Popliteus; Semitendinosus; Semimembranosus; Sartorius; Gracilis; Vastus Medialis

Lateral Rotation of Tibia on Femur
Biceps Femoris; Vastus Lateralis

Chapter

10

The Ankle Joint and Foot

The construction of the ankle joint/foot is most intriguing. The 26 bones (7 tarsals, 5 metatarsals and 14 phalanges), 19 large muscles, many small intrinsic muscles on the sole of the foot, and over 100 ligaments compose the main structure of **each** ankle joint and foot. The transfer of weight from the tibia, to the talus, to the calcaneus (heel bone) is an amazing balancing act while it accepts the weight of the entire body, and then propels it forward through the rest of the foot.

Joints and Actions of the Ankle Joint and Foot

The upper, or superior, ankle joint is the articulation point of the tibia, fibula, and talus. They fit together tightly; it is a true hinge joint where the actions of plantar and dorsiflexion take place. The lower, or inferior, ankle joint is a combination of the subtalar and the transverse tarsal joint. The seven tarsal bones are located within this area, and there is diverse movement between the various articulations. This author prefers to simplify the joint actions of the area, using the terms 'pronation' and 'supination' (see page 175).

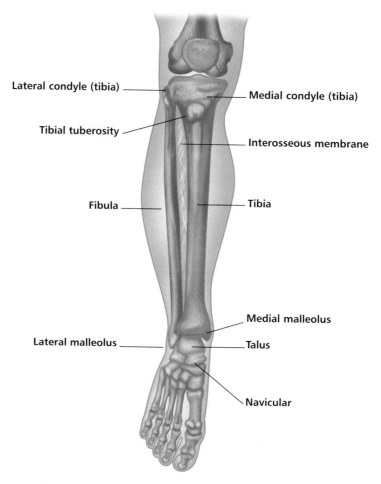

Lateral condyle (tibia)

Medial condyle (tibia)

Tibial tuberosity

Interosseous membrane

Fibula

Tibia

Medial malleolus

Lateral malleolus

Talus

Navicular

Figure 10.1: The right ankle joint/foot, anteromedial view.

There is a tarsal-metatarsal joint area that is called 'irregular', where gliding motion takes place. Some texts even refer to plantar and dorsiflexion as possible here. The joints are reinforced by many smaller ligaments.

The metatarsophalangeal joints can flex (dorsiflex), extend (plantar flex), and abduct, adduct, and rotate minimally. The interphalangeal joints flex and extend only. The proximal portion can only extend, the distal section can do both.

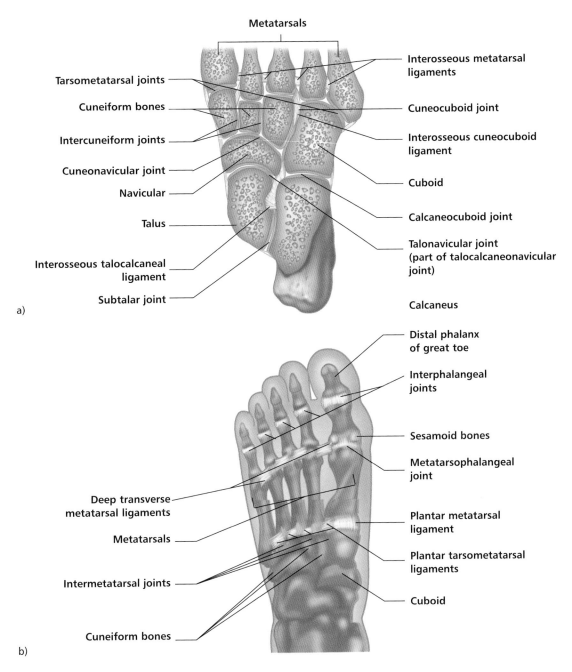

Figure 10.2: Joints of the foot, a) horizontal section of right foot, b) plantar view.

There is always some confusion over the terms used to describe actions of the ankle. To clarify, dorsiflexion is the act of 'flexing the foot', and plantar flexion is the act of 'pointing the foot', or extending. The joint is more stable in dorsiflexion. Pronation is a combination of eversion and abduction, where weight is placed on the medial side of the foot. Supination is a combination of inversion and adduction, where weight is on the outside, or lateral part of the foot. When the toes are flexed, they curl forward; when extended, they straighten.

The Anatomy of Exercise & Movement

The big toe, sometimes called the great toe, has larger bones than the other toes and is referred to as the hallux. It plays an important part in walking, running, even standing.

Muscles of the Ankle Joint and Foot

Extrinsic muscles of the foot are attached to the upper ankle bones of either the tibia or fibula. Two of them, the gastrocnemius and plantaris, even attach as high as the femur. Extrinsic muscles originate outside the body part they affect; proximally they attach above the foot, and then long tendons attach distally to the foot to work it. Intrinsic muscles are short muscles located on the sole of the foot, the plantar surface. Muscles of the ankle can be categorized by location:

1. Dorsiflexors are anterior
2. Plantar flexors are posterior
3. Pronators are mostly lateral
4. Supinators are either anterior, posterior (as in the tibialis anterior and the tibialis posterior) or on the plantar side of the foot
5. Toe flexors are posterior
6. Toe extensors are anterior

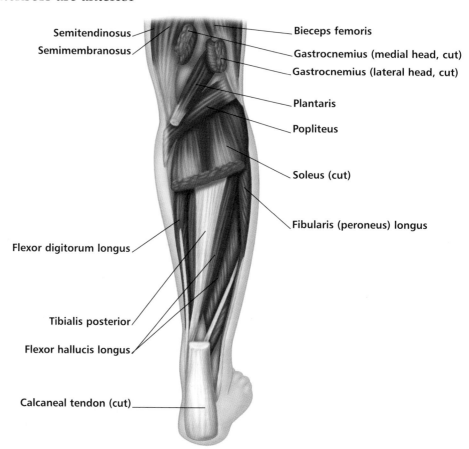

Figure 10.3: The calf muscles, right leg, posterior view.

At most other joints in the body the last two actions, flexion and extension, are reversed as far as location: flexor muscles are anterior and extensor muscles are posterior. There are three anterior muscles of the ankle/foot: **tibialis anterior, extensor digitorum longus, and extensor hallucis longus**. Each is a strong dorsiflexor, as well as the peroneus tertius, whose distal tendon appears anterior. These muscles also work the lower joints, making them bi- or multiarticulate.

The lateral muscles are considered the **peroneus tertius, longus, and brevis.** They all pronate, but the last two can also plantar flex.

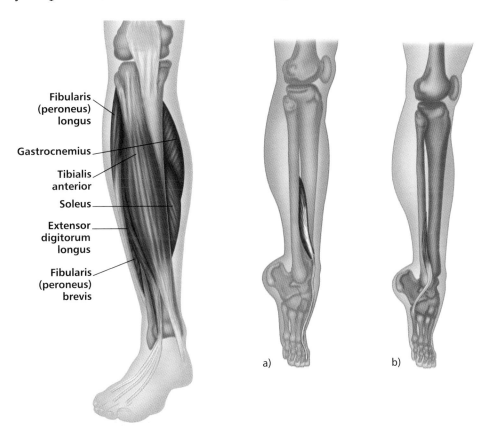

Figure 10.4: Superficial muscles of the lower leg (anterior view). Inset (a) extensor hallucis longus, (b) peroneus tertius.

There are six posterior muscles. The most commonly known are the **gastrocnemius** and the **soleus**. Identified as the calf muscle, the gastrocnemius gets its name from the Greek "gastroknemia", translated as 'belly of the calf'. Interestingly, the two proximal heads of the muscle are not on the lower leg, but above the knee. They attach to the femoral condyles in the back of the femur, and because they cross the knee joint, assist in flexion of the knee with the hamstrings. The most important action is at the ankle, where it crosses the joint by way of the strongest yet most injured tendon in the body, the Achilles. The gastrocnemius performs plantar flexion (pointing the foot). The soleus is a single joint muscle that helps shape the calf, and along with the gastrocnemius is known as the *triceps surae* (three heads, two muscles). Standing on the balls of the feet contracts and enhances this area, as plantar flexion of the ankle is performed. To stretch these muscles, dorsiflex the foot. To isolate the stretch of the gastrocnemius, also straighten the knee.

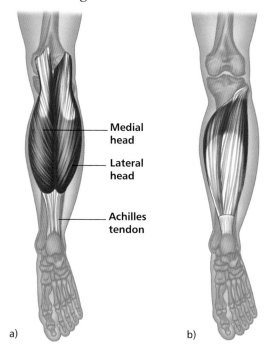

Figure 10.5: The two main posterior calf muscles; a) gastrocnemius, b) soleus.

The gastrocnemius is a 'fast mover', so very prominent in jumping, while the soleus can be defined as a *holding* muscle, working harder during a ballet releve or pointe work. As a biarticulate muscle, the gastrocnemius is stronger when it is working only one of its joints. It will plantar flex better if the knee is straight, and will bend the knee more if the ankle is dorsiflexed, especially if the foot is off the floor.

The gastrocnemius as the main mover of the ankle in jumping is concentrically contracting (shortening) on the way up, and eccentrically contracting (lengthening) on the landing. This means it is a main ankle muscle working throughout the jump.

Remember, muscles do not flex, joints do; muscles contract.

The **tibialis posterior** is a deep calf muscle. While it plantar flexes and supinates, it also supports the arches. The **plantaris** is a muscle that is biarticulate with the knee and ankle, but can only perform weak flexion at both joints.

Other posterior muscles are the **flexor digitorum longus** and **flexor hallucis longus**. The last is an important muscle in pointe work in ballet, as it aids balance while standing on tiptoe.

Calf Strengthening Exercises

Calf raises, jumping jacks or rope

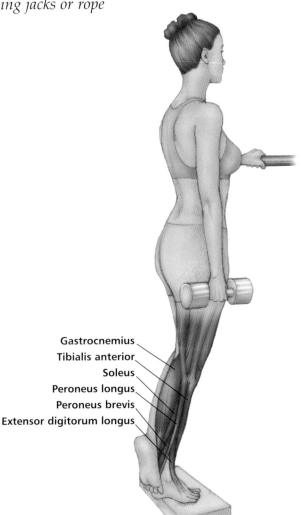

Gastrocnemius
Tibialis anterior
Soleus
Peroneus longus
Peroneus brevis
Extensor digitorum longus

Figure 10.6: Calf raises.

TECHNIQUE

With body vertical, place the ball joint to the toe of one or both feet on a step. Either one or both feet should be extended, so that the heel and arch of each foot is beyond the edge of the step. Hips, ankle(s), shoulders aligned, with spine in neutral position; head up. Use a dumbbell if you are using only one leg.

Calf Stretching Exercise

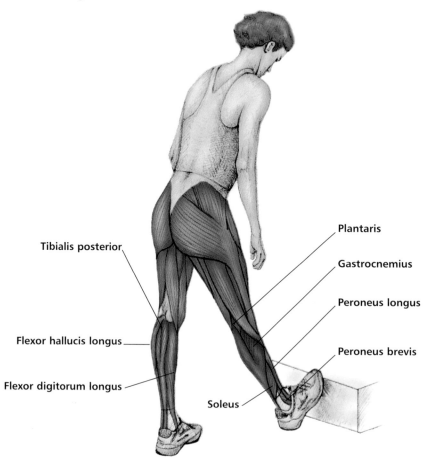

Tibialis posterior

Flexor hallucis longus

Flexor digitorum longus

Plantaris

Gastrocnemius

Peroneus longus

Peroneus brevis

Soleus

Figure 10.7: Standing toe-up calf stretch.

TECHNIQUE

Stand upright and place the toes on a step of raised object. Keep leg straight and lean toward toes.

The Foot

The arch-like construction of the foot makes it more than suited for the purposes of support, adaptability, absorbing shock, weight transfer, and propulsion. Five metatarsals form the instep or sole of the foot, and each toe has three phalanges, except the big toe, which has only two.

The arches are a lesson in architecture. Three arches form a "dome" to perform the necessary functions of the foot. The main longitudinal arch is on the medial side, consisting of the calcaneus on one side, four tarsals on the front side, with the talus in the middle acting as the 'keystone'. Laterally a longitudinal arch travels from the calcaneus through the talus to the cuboid and 4th and 5th metatarsals. The transverse arch crosses the foot from the big toe to the little toe metatarsal. The action of all lines of force is centered where the transverse and longitudinal arches meet, accepting weight from above and impact from below. Extrinsic muscles and those in the sole of the foot reinforce the arches. Put the two feet together parallel and there is a complete dome in the center of both.

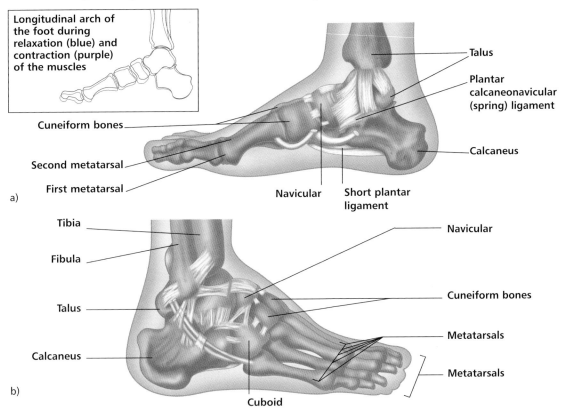

Figure 10.8: The arches of the foot; a) right foot, medial view, b) right foot, lateral view.

Ligaments of the Ankle Joint and Foot

The ligaments and tendons of the ankle joint/foot work together to support and maintain the position of the arches while connecting all 26 bones. The longest of all ligaments of the tarsals is the plantar ligament. It travels from the calcaneus, inserting on the cuboid bone, and extending to the 2nd, 3rd and 4th metatarsals. The plantar fascia is a broad structure that follows a similar path and supports the medial longitudinal arch.

The anterior and posterior talofibular ligaments run from the malleoli (outside points of the distal end of the fibula and tibia, easily seen), to the talus. The calcaneofibular ligament comes from the lateral malleolus and connects to the calcaneus. Medially, the large deltoid ligament runs from the medial malleolus to the talus and navicular. This ligament is so strong that in extreme, forceful pronation the bone can be fractured before the ligament tears.

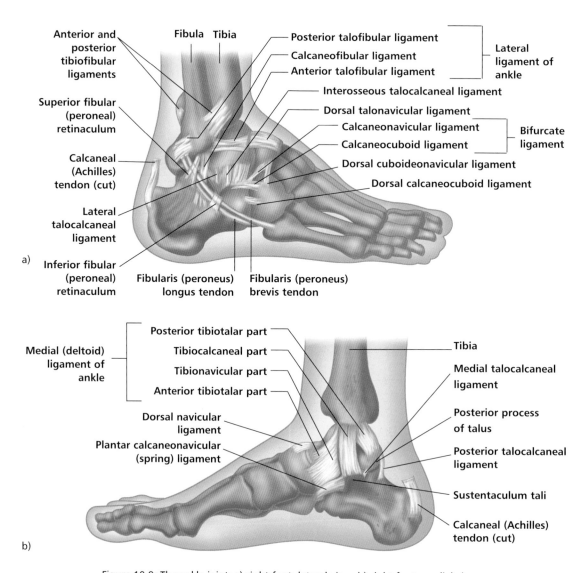

Figure 10.9: The ankle joint; a) right foot, lateral view, b) right foot, medial view.

Ankle Joint and Foot Conditions

Unwanted ankle joint/foot conditions appear from misalignment, misuse, or bad footwear (more on shoes later). Here are a few:

Bone Conditions

The medial arch is higher than the lateral because it works in motion, while the lateral supports more weight. The weight on the medial side transfers to the first metatarsal, a large bone that articulates with the big toe. Pressure here can lead to **bunions** or **bone spurs**, due to how the weight has been absorbed at this spot.
Corrections: Misalignment on impact can be corrected through weight distribution or better shoes, hopefully before surgery is needed.

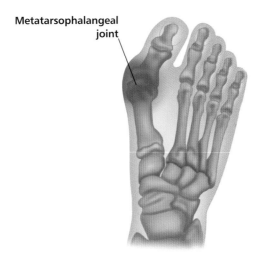

Metatarsophalangeal joint

Figure 10.10: Bunion and misalignment of big toe, caused primarlity by ill-fitting shoes.

A **stress fracture** (hairline bone fracture) can happen in the lower leg or foot bones and should be x-rayed by a physician. Actually, these can happen anywhere in the body, and are due to misalignment and overuse.

Muscle Conditions

Shin splints are a common injury in the lower leg caused by hard impact from the ground, up through the feet to the tibialis muscles. Anyone can get them, by walking or running on hard surfaces, landing incorrectly, or overuse. (Walking on concrete in heels is overuse for the lower leg muscles!) Muscle fibers can tear or begin to pull off the bone causing pain and inflammation.

Corrections: The only treatment is ice and rest; ankle exercises can be done once there is no pain.

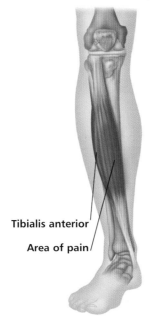

Tibialis anterior

Area of pain

Figure 10.11: Medial tibial pain syndrome (shin splints).

Connective Tissue Conditions

A thick layer of tough fibrous tissue, the plantar aponeurosis (or plantar fascia) travels from the calcaneus (heel bone) to the metatarsal heads (similar to the palmar aponeurosis in the hand). The plantar fascia helps support the arches of the foot, but can become inflamed, causing **plantar fasciitis**. This can be due to tight calves, high heels, flip-flops, activities that require a lot of footwork such as ballet or running, bad foot mechanics, or even obesity.

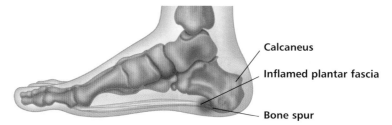

Calcaneus

Inflamed plantar fascia

Bone spur

Figure 10.12: Plantar fasciitis.

Corrections: Stretching exercises can be done for the Achilles tendon, the fascia, and muscles that support the lower leg (see figure 10.13), as well as some strength work. These cannot be overdone or the pain may persist. Orthotics can be used to help distribute pressure, prescribed by a therapist or doctor.

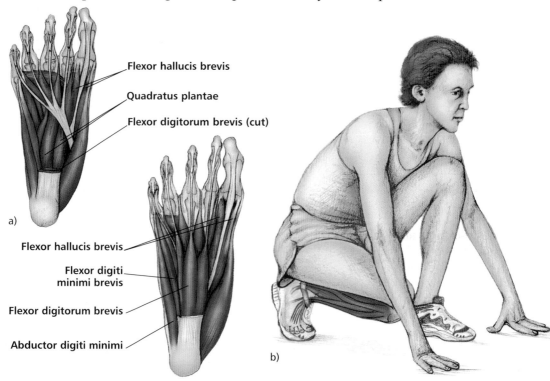

Flexor hallucis brevis

Quadratus plantae

Flexor digitorum brevis (cut)

a)

Flexor hallucis brevis

Flexor digiti minimi brevis

Flexor digitorum brevis

Abductor digiti minimi

b)

Figure 10.13: a) Right foot, plantar view, and b) squatting toe stretch.

TECHNIQUE

Kneel on one knee with hands on the ground. Place body weight over knee and slowly move knee forward. Keep toes on the ground and arch foot.

A most alarming fact is what people do to their feet. Scenarios:

1) The high heel is the worst possible shoe for balance and the Achilles tendon.
2) Plastic or rubber flip-flops are no better: there is no support, and ankle and knee conditions are becoming common.
3) Toes are squeezed into pointed tips and become cramped.

Wear a shoe that conforms to the shape of the foot while supporting it. If **pronation** is a problem (weight on the inside of the foot), wear a shoe that supports the medial inside arch. If **supination** is present (weight on the outside), use shoes that aid the lateral or outside of the foot. If not sure, look at a pair of shoes that have been exhausted by use, and see what side of the shoe is more worn. A good shoe salesman or physical therapist can also help determine the imbalance. **Good sneakers or well-made sandals can correct misalignment and help absorb shock from impact while exercising the muscles.**

Myths of the Foot Dispelled

A low arch is not necessarily a flat or weak foot
A low arch is common on the medial side, but if not weight-bearing, does not usually present a problem. However, 'fallen arches' can happen, caused by disuse or malfunction of the foot, and if painful, need treatment. A 'flat foot', which is typically an abnormality that is present since birth, can also be diagnosed. The methods used to help these conditions are orthotic inserts or correct shoes.

The medial arch does not bear weight, but if the muscles are not strong enough, the arch will weaken. The flexor hallucis longus is a muscle that flexes the big toe, but also stretches along this arch from the phalanges all the way to the fibula. Other muscles on the medial underside of the foot will also aid the arch. The three weight-bearing bones of the foot are the calcaneus, metatarsal 1 (the big toe, or hallux), and metatarsal 5 (the pinky), with many ligaments stabilizing them. **The full foot mechanism must be in balance and used properly to function correctly.**

A desired high arch might not be the ideal in all cases
While the foot is shaped nicely if there is a high medial and transverse arch, this can cause instability. Problems occur because:
1) Shoes may not fit very well because of the higher arch;
2) There may be some pain in the arch area because of pressure. Supination can occur. In the case of a ballet student, the high arch is desired, but ballet shoes and/or forced turn out can cause pronation.
Foot conditions can transfer up the body, causing problems in the shins, knee, hip and even the spine. Care must be taken with the feet to prevent injury

Shoes are not all the fashion industry has built them up to be
Rising up on the balls of the feet, as in a ballet releve or weight-room calf raise, can strengthen the feet, but remaining up (as in high heels) is detrimental. Staying flat in flip-flops, and on flat surfaces, is also contra-indicated.

The Anatomy of Exercise & Movement

Main Muscles Involved in Movements of the Ankle Joint and Foot

Dorsiflexion
Tibialis Anterior, Extensor Hallucis Longus; Extensor Digitorum Longus; Fibularis (Peroneus) Tertius

Plantar Flexion
Gastrocnemius; Plantaris; Soleus; Tibialis Posterior; Flexor Hallucis Longus; Flexor Digitorum Longus; Fibularis (Peroneus) Longus; Fibularis (Peroneus) Brevis

Intertarsal Joints

Inversion (supination)
Tibialis Anterior; Tibialis Posterior

Eversion (pronation)
Fibularis (Peroneus) Tertius; Fibularis (Peroneus) Longus; Fibularis (Peroneus) Brevis

Other Movements
Sliding movements, which allow some dorsiflexion, plantar flexion, abduction and adduction, are produced by the muscles acting on the toes. Tibialis Anterior, Tibialis Posterior, and Fibularis (Peroneus) Tertius are also involved.

Metatarsophalangeal Joints of the Toes

Flexion
Flexor Hallucis Brevis; Flexor Hallucis Longus; Flexor Digitorum Longus; Flexor Digitorum Brevis; Flexor Digiti Minimi Brevis; Lumbricales; Interossei

Extension
Extensor Hallucis Longus; Extensor Digitorum Brevis; Extensor Digitorum Longus

Abduction and Adduction
Abductor Hallucis; Adductor Hallucis; Interossei; Abductor Digiti Minimi

Interphalangeal Joints of the Toes

Flexion
Flexor Hallucis Longus; Flexor Digitorum Brevis (proximal joint only); Flexor Digitorum Longus

Extension
Extensor Hallucis Longus; Extensor Digitorum Brevis (not in great toe); Extensor Digitorum Longus; Lumbricales

The jawbone (mandible) articulates with the skull to form the **temporo-mandibular** joint; its muscles produce chewing. Another motion in eating is the grasping, or seizing of food by the powerful jaw muscles: the **temporalis, masseter**, and **pterygoids**. They open, shut, and grind the teeth, an occurrence that stress produces, sometimes during sleep.

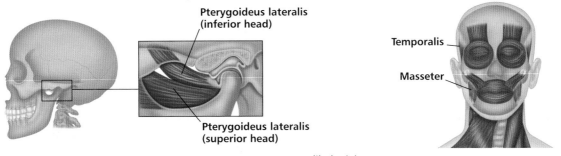

Figure A1: Temporo-mandibular joint.

Temporo-mandibular Joint Dysfunction

This is a dysfunction of the jaw joint and prevalent today, in many cases because of stress. Tension can misalign the placement of the jaw and impinge on nerves, leading to more problems and possible surgery. Keep in mind this is not the only reason for TMJ dysfunction; there could be bony limitations or other causes. Correct alignment is once again the key.

The Voice

Inside the throat area is the 'voice box', or **larynx**, which houses the vocal cords. This is suspended from the skull by a complicated system of muscles, and with the thyroid and pharynx travels toward the trachea and esophagus. I will not begin to explain this whole mechanism; it is beyond the scope of this book and my knowledge. Since my daughter is a singer, I will mention two related regions, the tongue area and palate.

The **tongue** is a muscle that has a system of extrinsic (outside) muscles that allow it to move in all directions. The intrinsic muscles are fibers within the tongue that move its tip to help speak, position food, and clean teeth. The tongue is connected to the hyoid bone above the larynx in the back of the throat. This connection is related to the operation of the larynx, and even head balance. When the tongue is relaxed on the floor of the mouth, there is less tension in the jaw and throat, which leads to a stronger voice.

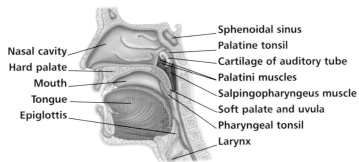

Figure A2: Sagittal section of nasal cavity.

The **palate** is the roof of the mouth. The hard palate is in front, the soft palate behind. Vocal teachers talk about "lifting the palate" to open the throat and produce a clearer sound. This is done by small but important muscles called the **palatines** and **salpingopharyngeus**; using these muscles helps resonance, and can be found by looking at the soft palate while yawning, and felt when humming.

References

1. Biel, A.: 2001. *Trail Guide to the Body, 2e*. Books of Discovery, Boulder, USA

2. Calais-Germain, B.: 2007. *Anatomy of Movement, Revised Edition*. Eastland Press, Seattle, USA

3. Clippinger, K.S.: 2006. *Dance Anatomy & Kinesiology*. Human Kinetics, Champaign, USA

4. Coulter, D. H.: 2001. *Anatomy of Hatha Yoga*. Body and Breath, New York, USA

5. Delavier, F.: 2006. *Strength Training Anatomy, 2e*. Human Kinetics, Champaign, USA

6. Dimon, T.: 2001. *Anatomy of the Human Body*. North Atlantic Books, Berkeley, USA

7. Egoscue, P.: 2000. *Pain Free: A Revolutionary Method for Stopping Chronic Pain*. Bantam Books, London, UK

8. Fitt, S. S.: 1996. *Dance Kinesiology*. Schirmer Books, New York, USA

9. Floyd, R.T. & Thompson, C.W.: 2009. *Manual of Structural Kinesiology, 17e*. McGraw-Hill, New York, USA

10. Franklin, E.: 2003. *Pelvic Power*. Princeton Book Company, New Jersey, USA

11. Hamilton, N., Weimar, W. & Luttgens, K.: 2007. *Kinesiology: Scientific Basis of Human Motion*. McGraw-Hill, New York, USA

12. Jarmey, C.: 2006. *The Concise Book of the Moving Body*. Lotus Publishing, Chichester, UK/North Atlantic Books, Berkeley, USA

13. Jarmey, C.: 2008. *The Concise Book of Muscles, 2e*. Lotus Publishing, Chichester, UK/North Atlantic Books, Berkeley, USA

14. Kaminoff, L.: 2007. *Yoga Anatomy*. Human Kinetics, Champaign, USA

15. Koch, L.: 2001. *The Psoas Book*. Guinea Pig Publications, Felton, USA

16. Long, R.: 2006. *The Key Muscles of Hatha Yoga*. Bandha Yoga Publications, New York, USA

17. Manocchia, P.: 2007. *Anatomy of Exercise*. A & C Black, London, UK

18. Massey, P.: 2009. *The Anatomy of Pilates*. Lotus Publishing, Chichester, UK/North Atlantic Books, Berkeley, USA

19. Mehta, S., Mehta, M. & Mehta, S.: 1990. *Yoga: the Iyengar Way*. Knopf, New York, USA

20. Niel-Asher, S.: 2008. *The Concise Book of Trigger Points, 2e*. Lotus Publishing, Chichester, UK/North Atlantic Books, Berkeley, USA

21. Norris, C. M.: 1998. *Sports Injuries: Diagnosis and Management*. Butterworth-Heinemann, Oxford, UK

22. Siler, B.: 2000. *The Pilates Body*. Broadway Books, New York, USA

23. Stone, R.J. & Stone, J.A.: *Atlas of Skeletal Muscles, 3e*. McGraw-Hill, New York, USA

24. Todd, M.E.: 1980. *The Thinking Body*. Princeton Book Company, New Jersey, USA

25. Vella, M.: 2008. *Anatomy for Strength & Fitness Training*. New Holland, Cape Town, South Africa

26. Walker, B.: 2007. *The Anatomy of Stretching*. Lotus Publishing, Chichester, UK/North Atlantic Books, Berkeley, USA

27. Walker, B.: 2008. *The Anatomy of Sports Injuries*. Lotus Publishing, Chichester, UK/North Atlantic Books, Berkeley, USA

28. Wharton, J. & Wharton, P.: 1996. *Stretch Book*. Times Books, New York, USA

29. Wilmore, J.H. & Costill, D.L.: 1994. *Physiology of Sport & Exercise*. Human Kinetics, Champaign, USA

Index

General Index

Abduction 10
Acetabulum 72
Acetylcholine 18
Acromion process 82
Actin 16, 19
Action potential 18
Adduction 10
Adenosine triphosphate
(ATP) 19
Agonist 20, 127
'All or nothing principle' 17
Amphiarthrotic joints, *see slightly moveable joints*
Anatomical position 16
Anisotropic (A) bands 16
Ankle joint 173
Annular ligament
of radius 108
Antagonist 20, 127
Anterior 8
Anterior cruciate
ligament 167
Anterior tibial translation 167
Aponeurosis 17
Atlanto-axial joint 30
Atlanto-occipital joint 30
Attachments 20

Ball-and-socket joints 26
Bone spurs 182
Brachial plexus 117
Breastbone, *see sternum*
Breathing 24
Bunions 182
Bursae 25, 160

Carpals 121
Carpal tunnel syndrome 117
Cartilage 169
Chondromalacia patellae 169

Circular muscles 16
Circumduction 10
Collateral ligaments 170
Concentric
contractions 21, 49, 53
Contractions 20
Contralateral 8
Convergent muscles 16
Coracoid process 104
Coronal plane 9, 73
Cross-bridges 16

Deep 8
Depression 11
Diaphysis 41
Diarthrotic joints, *see freely moveable joints*
Distal 18
Dorsiflexion 12
Dorsum 8

Eccentric
contractions 22, 49, 53
Elbow joint 101
Elevation 11
Endomysium 15, 17
End plate potential 18
Epimysium 15, 17
Eversion 12
Extension 11
Extensor retinaculum 116

Fascia 15
Fasciculus 15
Flexor retinaculum 116
Flexion 11
Floating ribs 35
Foot 180
Force 23
Freely moveable joints 25
Frontal plane,
see coronal plane

Glenohumeral joint 78

Glenoid fossa 104
Glenoid labrum 78
Gliding joints,
see plane joints
Glycogen 14
Golfer's elbow,
see medial epicondylitis
Golgi tendon organs
(GTO's) 19

Hinge joints 26
Hip joint 123
Horizontal plane,
see transverse plane

Iliofemoral joint 70, 72, 123
Iliofemoral ligament 142
Ilio-tibial band 131
Ilium 69
Immoveable joints 25
Inferior 8
Insertions 20
Intermediate fast-twitch
fibers 14
Interphalangeal joint 114
Intra-abdominal pressure 24
Intrafusal fibers 19
Inversion 12
Ipsilateral 8, 50
Isometric
contractions 22, 49, 53
Isotropic (I) bands 16

Knee jerk test 20
Knee joint 159

Larynx 187
Latent potential 18
Lateral 8
Lateral epicondylitis 107
Lateral flexion 11
Levers 22
Ligaments 70, 79, 102, 160, 181
Lumbar vertebrae 48

Medial   8
Medial epicondylitis   108
Median plane   9, 73
Meniscus   170
Metacarpo-phalangeal
    joint   114
Metatarsals   173
Metatarso-phalangeal
    joints   175
Mid-sagittal plane,
    see median plane
Mobilizers   21
Motor nerve fiber   17
Motor unit   17
Multipennate muscles   82
Muscle contraction   18
Muscle reflexes   19
Muscle spindles   19
Musculo-skeletal
    mechanics   20
Myofibrils   16
Myofilaments   16
Myoglobin   14
Myosin   16, 19

Nerve endings   19
Neuromuscular junction   18

Opposition   8,115
Origin   20
Overloading   53

Palmar   8
Palmar aponeurosis   116
Parallel muscles   16
Pelvic floor muscles   25
Pelvic tilt   71
Pelvis   69
Pennate muscles   16
Perimysium   15, 17
Perineal center   74
Periosteum   17
Peripheral   8
Pilates   129

Pivot joints   26
Plane joints   26
Planes of the body   19
Plantar   8
Plantar fascia   184
Plantar flexion   12
Plyometrics   168
Posterior   8
Pranayamas   57
Prime mover,
    see agonist
Pronation   11, 108, 175
Prone   8
Proprioception   19
Protraction   12
Proximal   8

Q angle   163

Radio-ulnar joint   101, 108
Range of motion   59
Red slow-twitch fibers   124
Reposition   8
Resting potential   18
Retraction   12
Rotation   12
Rotator cuff   87
Runner's knee, see
    chondromalacia patellae

Sacro-iliac joint   70
Sacrum   69
Saddle joints   26
Sagittal plane,
    see median plane
Sarcolemma   15, 18
Sarcoplasmic
    reticulum   15, 18
Sciatica   152
Secondary movers,
    see assistant movers
Shin splints   183
Shoulder girdle joint   91
Skeletal muscle   13

Sliding filament theory   18
Slightly moveable joints   25
Squats   129
Stabilizers,   21,127
Static contraction, see
    isometric contraction
Sternoclavicular joint   91
Sternum   35
Stress fracture   183
Stretch reflex arc   20, 59
Stretching   59
Subacromial bursa   87
Superficial   8
Superior   8
Supination   11, 108, 175
Supine   8
Synaptic terminals   18
Synarthrotic joints,
    see immoveable joints
Synergist   20, 63
Synovial joints   25

Tarsals   173
Temporo-mandibular
    joint   187
Tendonitis   104
Tennis elbow,
    see lateral epicondylitis
Titin   16
Tongue   187
Transverse plane   9, 10, 73
Transverse (T) tubules   15
Triceps surae   178

Ulnar tunnel syndrome   118
Unipennate muscles   132
Uterus   244

Vertebral column   29

White fast-twitch fibers   14

Index of Muscles

Adductor brevis 147
Adductor longus 147
Adductor magnus 147
Anconeus 103

Biceps
  brachii 81, 103, 104, 109
Biceps femoris 144, 165
Brachialis 103
Brachioradialis 103, 109

Coracobrachialis 81

Deltoids 81
Diaphragm 24

Erector spinae 31, 36
Extensor carpi
  radialis brevis 117
Extensor carpi
  radialis longus 117
Extensor carpi ulnaris 117
Extensor digitorum
  longus 177
Extensor hallucis longus 177
External obliques 54

Flexor carpi radialis 117
Flexor carpi ulnaris 117
Flexor digitorum longus 178
Flexor hallucis longus 178

Gastrocnemius 165, 177
Gemellus inferior 152
Gemellus superior 152
Gluteus maximus 139
Gluteus medius 132
Gluteus minimus 133
Gracilis 148, 165

Iliacus 165, 177
Iliopsoas 63, 126
Infraspinatus 81, 87
Internal obliques 56

Latissimus dorsi 81, 86
Levator scapulae 31
Longus capitis 31
Longus colli 31

Masseter 187

Obliquus capitis 31
Obturator externus 153
Obturator internus 152

Pectineus 147
Pectoralis major 81, 84
Peroneus brevis 177
Peroneus longus 177
Peroneus tertius 177
Piriformis 70, 152
Plantaris 165, 178
Popliteus 165
Pronator quadratus 109
Pronator teres 103, 109
Psoas major 63, 126
Psoas minor 63, 126
Pterygoids 187

Quadratus femoris 153
Quadratus lumborum 64, 68

Rectus abdominis 49
Rectus capitis anterior 31
Rectus femoris 124, 162
Rhomboids 37

Sartorius 125, 165
Scalenes 31
Semimembranosus 144, 165
Semispinalis 31, 36
Semitendinosus 144, 165
Soleus 177
Spleni 31
Sternocleidomastoid 31
Subscapularis 87
Supinator 109

Supraspinatus 87
Temporalis 187
Tensor fasciae latae 131
Teres major 81
Teres minor 81, 87
Tibialis anterior 177
Tibialis posterior 178
Transversus abdominis 57
Trapezius 31, 37, 93
Triceps brachii 81, 103, 105

Vastus intermedius 162
Vastus lateralis 162
Vastus medialis 162

Index of Exercises

Adho mukha svanasana
  (down dog) 40, 119
Adho mukha vrksasana
  (handstand) 119
Advanced inversions 33

Backbend 62
Back extension 42
Baddha konasana
  (butterfly pose) 150
Barbell plié squat 163
Behind the back
  chest stretch 120
Bench press 85
Bent arm chest stretch 85
Bent arm circles 98
Bent arm shoulder stretch 83
Bent-over lateral raises 89
Bhujangasana
  (cobra pose) 39
Biceps curl 110
Bottom leg lifts 148

Cable adduction 149
Cat 38/39
Child's pose 87, 142
Crossed leg stretch 138

Dhanurasana (bow pose)   67
Diagonal thigh cross   137
Dips   96
Dog (cow)   38/39
Dumbbell press   89
Dumbbell standing lateral
    raise   83

Elbow-out rotator stretch   90
Extensions   90

Garudasana (eagle pose)   111
Good mornings   42, 145

Half-bridge   60
Happy baby   74

Karate kicks   138
Kneeling back rotation
    stretch   43
Kneeling reach forward
    stretch   87

Lateral raises   88
Lat. pull downs   86
Leg abduction   135
Leg extensions
    to the back   67
Leg lowers   52
L-position   66
Leg presses   141
Lying leg curls   145

Machine adduction   149
Matsyasana (fish pose)   41

Parivrtta trikonasana
    (rotated triangle pose)   61
Partial sit-up   51
Paschimottanasana
    (seated forward bend)   143
Pilates criss-cross   55
Pilates double leg kicks   166
Pilates 100   34, 52
Pilates open leg rocker   44

Pilates saw   55
Pilates side circles with
    rotation   134
Pilates single leg kicks   145
Pilates spine stretch   41
Pilates swan   67
Pilates swan dive   131
Piriformis stretch   138
Posterior leg lifts   130, 141
Psoas lift   67
Pull-ups   111
Purvottanasana (upward
    plank pose)   97

Reaching upper
    back stretch   95
Rising stomach stretch   58
Roman chair roational
    crunches   56
Rond de jambe   154

Sacro-iliac joint strength   71
Sacro-iliac joint stretch   71
Salabhasana (locust pose)   39
Setu bandha
    (bridge pose)   129, 141
Side-bending   51
Side leg press   135
Side stretches   98
Sitting abduction   132
Sitting adduction   148
Sitting foot-to-chest
    buttocks stretch   155
Sitting/lying leg rotation   154
Sitting side reach stretch   43
Sitting wide leg stretch   150
Spinal twists   60, 61
Standing lateral
    side reach   68
Standing leg rotation   154
Standing leg-up stretch   151
Standing toe-raised
    hamstring stretch   146
Standing toe-up
    calf stretch   180
Supine hip flexion   127

Supine spinal twists   142
Supine thigh cross   137
Swimming   62, 90, 148

Towel stretches   98
Turning wrist stretch   120
Twisting sit-ups   55

Upright rows   94
Upside-down butterfly   151
Urdhva mukha svanasana
    (up dog)   40
Ustrasana (camel pose)   131
Uttanasana (standing
    forward bend)   143

Virabhadrasana I
    (warrior pose)   130
Virabhadrasana II
    (warrior pose)   128
Vrksasana (tree pose)   136
V-seat   65

Weighted leg lifts   134
Windmills   54